Vegetaria

Cookbook

100+ Everyday Recipes for Beginners and Advanced Users. Try Easy and Healthy Vegetarian Diet Recipes

Inay Kumar

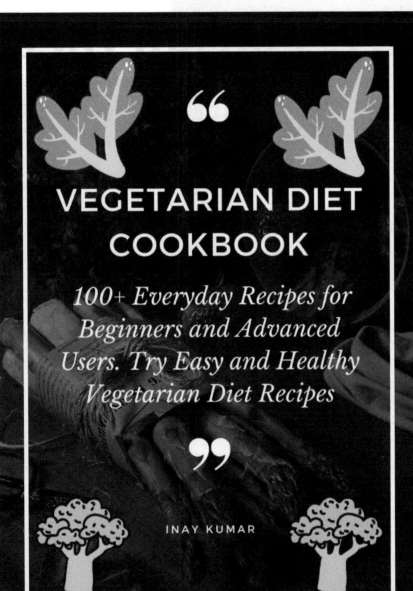

VEGETARIAN DIET COOKBOOK

100+ Everyday Recipes for Beginners and Advanced Users. Try Easy and Healthy Vegetarian Diet Recipes

INAY KUMAR

Table of Contents

INTRODUCTION

"Eating vegetarian 'is no longer the polarizing concept it once was, and it's not just full-time vegetarians who are interested in plant-based meals. There's ever-growing evidence of the benefits of eating fewer animal products. For others, environmental or political beliefs drive their choice.

But there are many reasons why you may choose to prepare a vegetarian recipe, even just occasionally. Maybe you're baking a birthday cake for a loved one. Maybe you want to add more whole grains and vegetarian to your diet, so you try eating vegetarian once a week, or for a month. Or maybe you're simply intrigued by the ingredients and flavors in vegetarian cuisine. We were, and that's why we've published our first vegetarian cookbook, one that suits the needs of everyone— whether you're a strict vegetarian or not. In doing so, we developed recipes (with no animal products — period) that wowed us in terms of flavor and texture, showing that veganism isn't about making sacrifices or substitutions but about celebrating a new way to eat. To be perfectly honest with you: vegetarianism is the most hardcore dieting imaginable. It can be mentally and emotionally exhausting to feel deprived of all the juicy processed foods, so this diet definitely isn't for beginners. Another challenge is adapting this kind of diet to your lifestyle while still keeping its core tenets intact. As soon as you start a vegetarian diet, you'll realize why carbs are so popular: they're easy to make, handle transport well and taste great. So, unless you have your logistics down to a science, you'll find it very difficult to maintain a vegetarian diet, but you should try it nonetheless and keep trying until you make it.

In the absence of certain food items, the vegetarian diet has also proved to be effective in stabilizing blood sugar. This diet has been linked to improving blood sugar levels in diabetic patients. The recipes covered here will help you live a healthy and fulfilling lifestyle.

More importantly, relax and enjoy the transformation in your life. That's another way to keep your new diet regimen sustainable. Your journey starts in the supermarket as you choose the best ingredients for your meals, and you can consider it an adventure. Try a new ingredient or spice. Enjoy the methods of preparation, savor the flavor and aroma of each dish, and keep on experimenting until you come up with the right flavors. More doable in the vegetarian diet as opposed to a general low-calorie diet.

If there is one drawback of the vegetarian diet, it's the sudden change in your temperament as you go through the transition period. Animal products leave a residue in your digestive system, which could lead you a bit depressed because it rigs your hormones. To help you detoxify gently, you can flush out toxins with lots of water. Squeeze in lemon juice from time to time for flavor and a kick of vitamin C.

On a more positive note, vegetarian diets can be good for the heart. Vegetarian diets can help decrease triglycerides levels and bad cholesterol in the bloodstream, which is why it is speculated that a vegetarian diet may soon trump the Mediterranean diet where heart health is concerned.

BREAKFAST

1. <u>PARMESAN PUFFS</u>

Preparation Time: 10 minutes

Cooking Time: 6 minutes

Servings: 12

INGREDIENTS

- 1/8 teaspoon salt

- 1 teaspoon basil, dried

- 4 organic egg, whites

- ½ cup Parmesan cheese, grated

- ½ cup olive oil for frying

DIRECTIONS

1. Add egg whites in a mixing bowl and whip until stiff peaks form. Gently fold basil, cheese, salt and egg whites. In a saucepan over medium heat add oil, when oil is hot adding a tablespoon of egg mix and cook for 3 minutes then turn over and cook on another side for 3 minutes. Serve warm and enjoy!

NUTRITION VALUES: Calories: 118 Fat: 11.1 g Carbohydrates: 0.8 g Sugar: 0.1 g Protein: 5.2 g Cholesterol: 10 mg

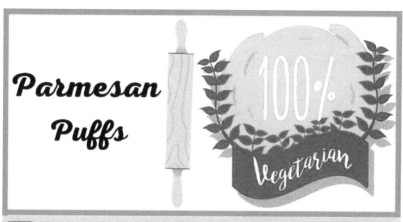

Parmesan Puffs

100% Vegetarian

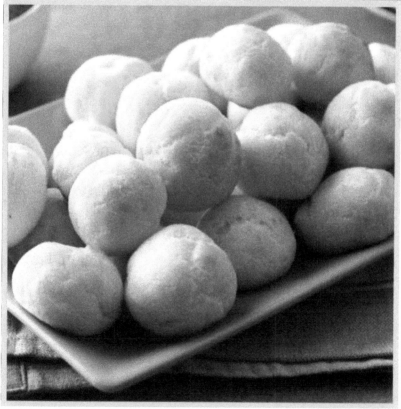

2. CHEESE & SPINACH EGG BREAKFAST

Preparation Time: 10 minutes

Cooking Time: 25 minutes

Servings: 4

INGREDIENTS

- 3 eggs, organic
- 3-ounces cottage cheese
- 4-ounces spinach, chopped
- ¼ cup Parmesan cheese, grated
- ¼ cup milk

DIRECTIONS

1. Preheat your oven to 375°Fahrenheit. Add half of Parmesan cheese, milk, eggs and cottage cheese in a mixing bowl. Whisk ingredients well. Add in the spinach and mix. In a greased baking dish pour your mixture into it. Sprinkle your remaining Parmesan cheese on top. Bake in your preheated oven for 25 minutes. Serve warm and enjoy!

NUTRITION VALUES: Calories: 145 Fat: 8.6 g Carbohydrates: 2.8 g Sugar: 1.1 g Protein: 14.4 g Cholesterol: 136 mg

Cheese & Spinach Egg Breakfast

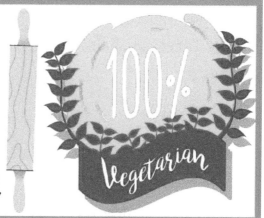

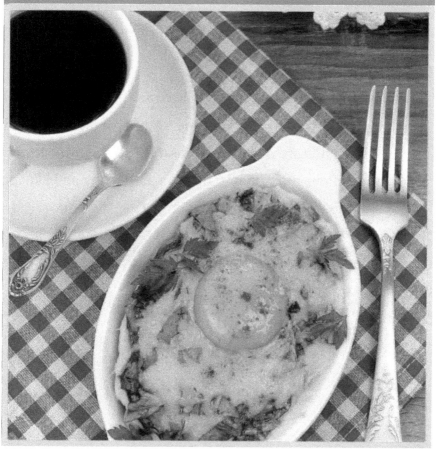

3. PARMESAN BREAKFAST CASSEROLE

Preparation Time: 5 minutes

Cooking Time: 25 minutes

Servings: 3

INGREDIENTS

- 5 eggs, organic

- 3 tablespoons tomato sauce, chunky

- 2 tablespoons heavy cream

- 2 tablespoons Parmesan cheese, grated, fresh

DIRECTIONS

1. Preheat your oven to 350° Fahrenheit. In a mixing bowl mix eggs and cream together. Add tomato sauce and cheese and mix well. Spray casserole dish with cooking spray. Pour mixture into the prepared dish and bake for 25 minutes. Serve warm and enjoy!

NUTRITION VALUES: Calories: 186 Fat: 14 g Carbohydrates: 1.7 g Sugar: 1.2 g Protein: 13.6 g Cholesterol: 293 mg

Parmesan Breakfast Casserole

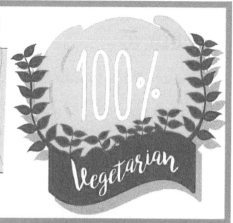

100%
Vegetarian

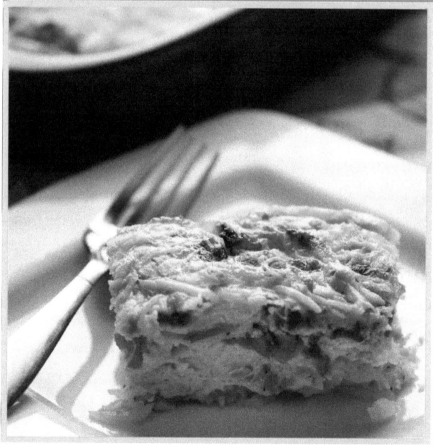

4. HEALTHY CHIA BANANA BREAKFAST PUDDING

Preparation Time: 10 minutes

Servings: 3

INGREDIENTS

- 1 medium banana, mashed
- 1 can full-fat coconut milk
- ½ teaspoon salt
- ½ teaspoon ground cinnamon
- 1 teaspoon vanilla extract
- ¼ cup chia seeds

DIRECTIONS

1. Add all your chia pudding ingredients into a mixing bowl and mix well. Place the mixing bowl in your fridge overnight. Serve in the morning and enjoy!

NUTRITION VALUES: Calories: 153 Fat: 10.4 g Carbohydrates: 17.8 g Sugar: 5 g Protein: 4.8 g Cholesterol: O mg

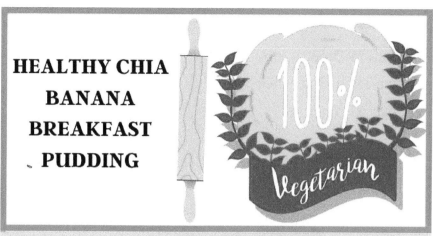

HEALTHY CHIA BANANA BREAKFAST PUDDING

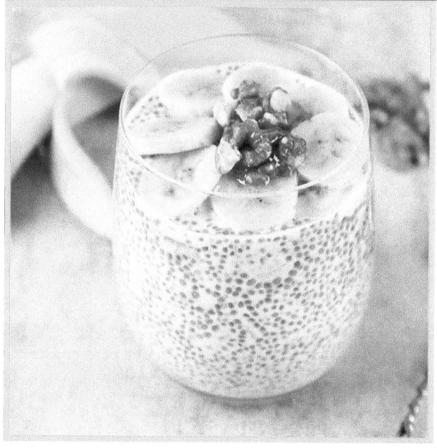

5. **<u>VEGGIE MIX OMELET</u>**

Preparation Time: 5 minutes

Cooking Time: 8 minutes

Servings: 4

INGREDIENTS

- ½ cup olives, bell pepper, onions
- ½ teaspoon parsley, chopped
- 1/2 cup spinach, finely chopped
- 3 eggs, organic
- Black pepper
- Olive oil for frying

DIRECTIONS

1. In a frying pan cover bottom with olive oil and heat over medium heat. Once the oil is heated, add the mixed veggies and stir-fry them. Once they are stir-fried remove from heat and set aside. In a mixing bowl, whisk eggs with pepper and 1 tablespoon water. Heat pan over medium heat. Spray pan with cooking spray. Pour egg mixture into the hot pan and cook your omelet, once it is cooked top with veggies and flip omelet to heat through. Serve hot and enjoy!

NUTRITION VALUES: Calories: 110 Fat: 6.6 g Carbohydrates: 3.3 g Sugar: 1.3 g Protein: 8.8 g Cholesterol: 246 mg

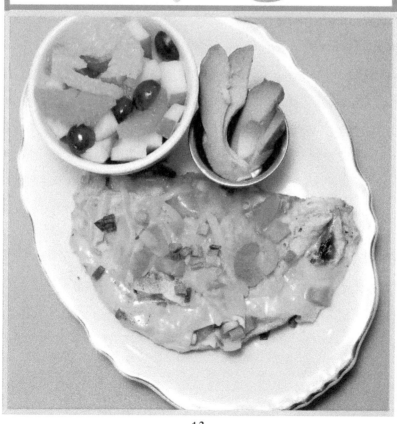

6. CINNAMON CREAM EGG PORRIDGE

Preparation Time: 5 minutes

Cooking Time: 5 minutes

Servings: 2

INGREDIENTS

- 1/3 cup heavy cream
- 2 eggs, organic
- 1/8 teaspoon cinnamon
- 2 tablespoons butter
- 2 single packages of Stevia

DIRECTIONS

1. In a mixing bowl, blend heavy cream, eggs, and Stevia. Melt butter in a saucepan over medium heat. Once your butter has melted reduce the heat to medium-low. Add egg and cream mixture into the saucepan and cook until it thickens. When it begins to curdle remove the pan from heat. Pour porridge into the serving bowl. Sprinkle the top of porridge with cinnamon. Serve and enjoy!

NUTRITION VALUES: Calories: 234 Fat: 23.3 g Carbohydrates: 1 g Sugar: 0.4 g Protein: 6.1 g Cholesterol: 222 mg

CINNAMON CREAM EGG PORRIDGE

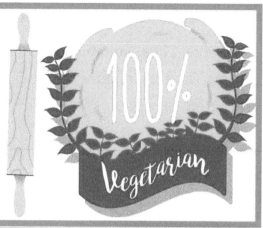

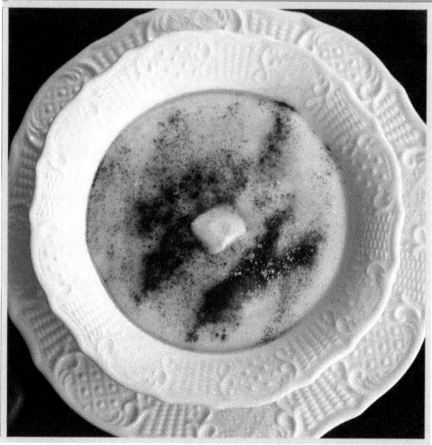

7. <u>CHEESY SQUASH BREAKFAST CASSEROLE</u>

Preparation Time: 10 minutes

Cooking Time: 25 minutes

Servings: 6

INGREDIENTS

- 12 organic eggs, beaten
- Salt and pepper
- 2 cups spaghetti squash, cooked
- 1 cup heavy cream
- 1 cup cheddar cheese, shredded
- ½ cup bell pepper, diced
- 4 tablespoons butter, melted

DIRECTIONS

1. Preheat your oven to 350°Fahrenheit. Take your baking dish and spray it with cooking spray and set aside.
2. In a mixing bowl, add all ingredients and mix well until combined.
3. Pour mixture into the prepared baking dish. In your preheated oven bake for 25 minutes or until done.
4. Allow cooling then you can serve and enjoy!

NUTRITION VALUES: Calories: 435 Fat: 37 g Carbohydrates: 5 g Sugar: 1.3 g Protein: 18.56 g Cholesterol: 395 mg

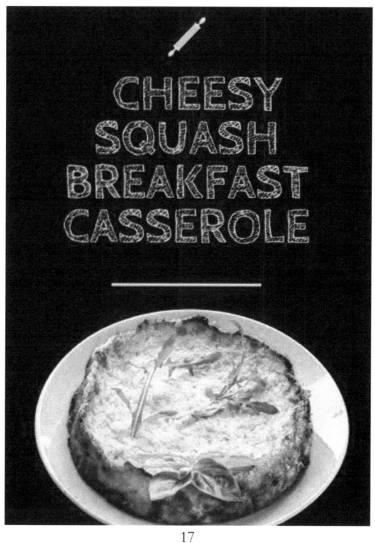

8. CHOCO BUTTER BREAKFAST SHAKE

Preparation Time: 10 minutes

Servings: 2

INGREDIENTS

- 2 tablespoons peanut butter, unsweetened
- 4 drops Stevia, liquid
- ½ cup coconut milk, unsweetened
- 2 scoops vanilla protein powder
- 2 tablespoons coconut oil

DIRECTIONS

1. Add all your ingredients into your blender and blend until smooth. Serve and enjoy!

NUTRITION VALUES: Calories: 467 Fat: 35 g Carbohydrates: 5.49 g Sugar: 3.1 g Protein: 30.45 g Cholesterol: 0 mg

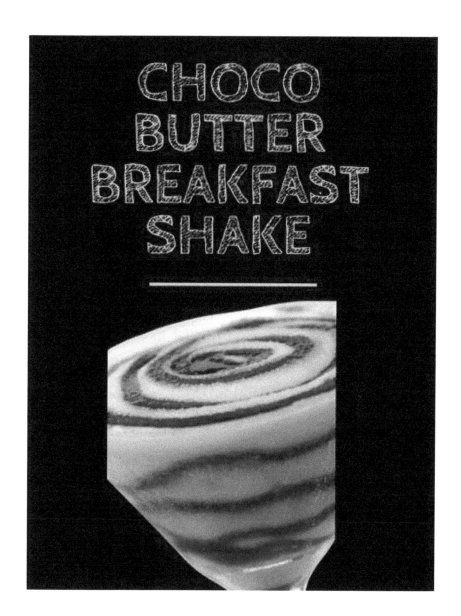

CHOCO BUTTER BREAKFAST SHAKE

9. SIMPLE BAKED EGG

Preparation Time: 5 minutes

Cooking Time: 15 minutes

Servings: 1

INGREDIENTS

- 1 large organic egg
- Salt and pepper
- 1 tablespoon heavy cream
- 1 teaspoon parsley, chopped
- 1 teaspoon chives, chopped
- ½ teaspoon butter

DIRECTIONS

1. Preheat your oven to 350°Fahrenheit. Grease ramekin with ½ teaspoon of butter. Crack an egg into a greased ramekin. Add heavy cream over egg then sprinkle chopped chives, parsley, salt, and pepper on top. Place ramekin into the oven and bake for 15 minutes. Serve and enjoy!

NUTRITION VALUES: Calories: 173 Fat: 15.7 g Carbohydrates: 0.5 g Sugar: 0.4 g Protein: 6.4 g Cholesterol: 221 mg

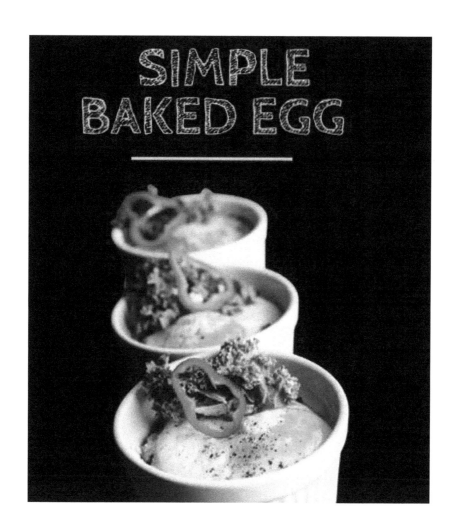

SIMPLE
BAKED EGG

10. <u>CREAMY ORANGE BREAKFAST SHAKE</u>

Preparation Time: 10 minutes

Servings: 4

INGREDIENTS

- 1 teaspoon orange extract
- 1 cup ice cubes
- 8-ounces cream cheese
- 1 ¼ cups almond milk, unsweetened
- ¼ cups almond
- ¼ teaspoon Stevia, powder
- 1 teaspoon vanilla

DIRECTIONS

1. Add all your ingredients into your blender and blend until smooth. Serve and enjoy!

NUTRITION VALUES: Calories: 213 Fat: 20.6 g Carbohydrates: 2.1 g Sugar: 0.4 g Protein: 4.6 g Cholesterol: 62 mg

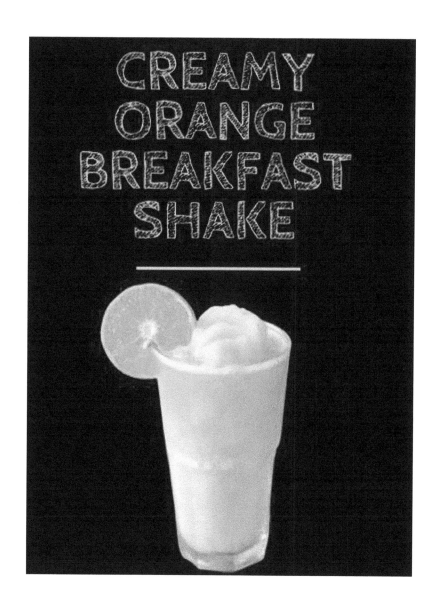

11. MINT ALMOND BREAKIE SHAKE

Preparation Time: 10 minutes

Servings: 2

INGREDIENTS

- 2 teaspoons mint extract
- 1 cup ice cubes
- 1 cup vanilla almond milk, unsweetened
- 4-ounces cream cheese
- ½ cup mint leaves
- ½ teaspoon Stevia, liquid

DIRECTIONS

1. Add all your ingredients into your blender and blend until smooth. Serve and enjoy!

NUTRITION VALUES: Calories: 238 Fat: 21 g Carbohydrates: 4 g Sugar: 0.6 g Protein: 8.5 g Cholesterol: 62 mg

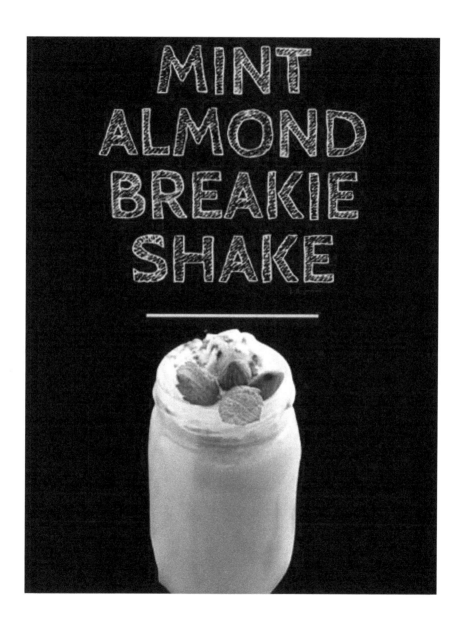

12. ENGLISH MUFFIN

Preparation Time: 10 minutes

Cooking Time: 1 minute

Servings: 1

INGREDIENTS

- 1 tablespoon Parmesan cheese, grated
- 1 teaspoon butter
- 1 large organic egg
- 2 teaspoons coconut flour
- 1/8 teaspoon baking soda
- 1/8 teaspoon sea salt

DIRECTIONS

1. Grease ramekin with butter and set aside. In a small bowl, combine egg and coconut flour. Now add all remaining ingredients, mix well. Place dough into prepared ramekin. Place ramekin into the microwave and microwave for I minute. Allow cooling for 5 minutes. Slice muffin in half and serve.

NUTRITION VALUES: Calories: 200 Fat: 14.3 g Carbohydrates: 4.4 g Sugar: 0.9 g Protein: 13.3 g Cholesterol: 206 mg

ENGLISH MUFFIN

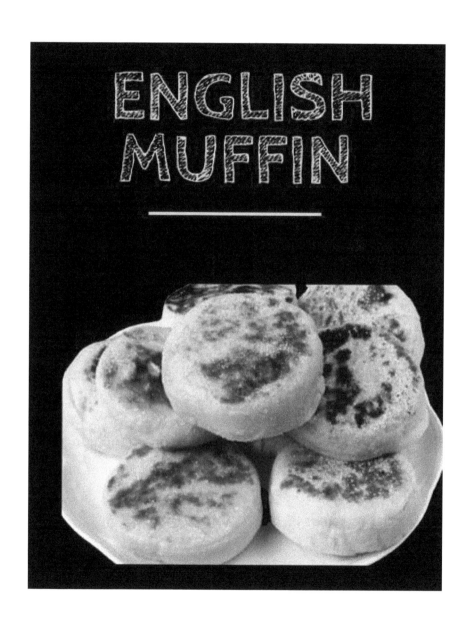

13. CHOCO BREAKFAST PUDDING

Preparation Time: 10 minutes

Cooking Time: 5 minutes

Servings: 4

INGREDIENTS

- 1 teaspoon vanilla extract

- 1/8 teaspoon sea salt

- 2 cups full fat coconut milk, divided

- ½ cup cocoa powder, unsweetened

- 1 tablespoon powdered gelatin

- 1 cup almond milk, unsweetened

- ½ teaspoon Stevia powder

DIRECTIONS

1. Add gelatin and ¼ cup coconut milk in a mixing bowl, stir well and set aside. Add remaining coconut milk in a saucepan and heat for 5 minutes or until hot. Pour almond milk into microwave safe bowl and microwave for 1 minute. Add cocoa powder and stevia into gelatin and mix well. Pour almond milk and coconut milk into gelatin mixture and stir continuously. Add vanilla extract and salt. Pour batter into the four serving cups and place in fridge until they set. Serve and enjoy!

NUTRITIONAL VALUES (Per Serving): Calories: 392 Fat: 36 g Carbohydrates: 13 g Sugar: 5 g Protein: 10 g Cholesterol: 0 mg

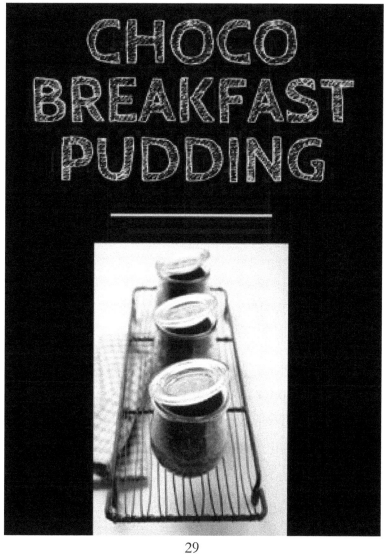

MAINS

14. ROASTED ARTICHOKES WITH WINE IN FOIL

Servings: 6

INGREDIENTS

- 6 stemmed globe artichokes
- ¼ c. olive oil
- 1 c. dry white wine
- 2 tbsps. Dried oregano
- 3 tsps. Chili flakes
- 2 chopped garlic cloves
- Kosher salt
- Black pepper

DIRECTIONS

1. Preheat oven to 450°F.
2. Cut top of each artichoke and pull leaves apart to open artichokes. Place artichokes in a greased baking dish.
3. Whisk together oil, wine, oregano, chili flakes, garlic, and salt and pepper in a bowl.
4. Pour the oil/wine mixture over each artichoke evenly.
5. Cover with aluminum foil, and bake for 45 minutes.
6. Uncover, and bake about 15 - 20 minutes more.
7. Let cool for 10 minutes before serving.

NUTRITION VALUES: Calories: 162.78 Fat: 7.47g Carbs: 7.12g Protein: 4.47g

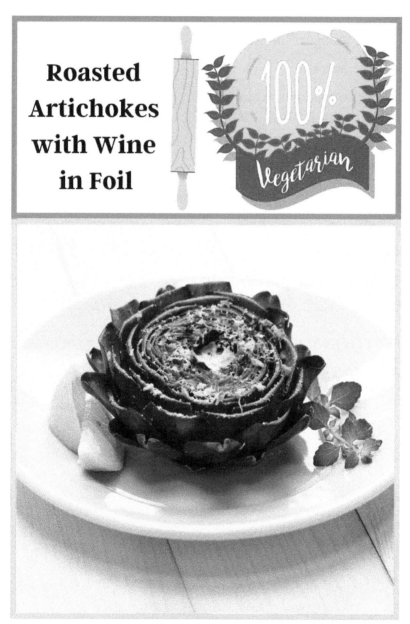

Roasted Artichokes with Wine in Foil

100% Vegetarian

15. <u>SOUR MARINATED CHAMPIGNONS</u>

Servings: 6

INGREDIENTS

- 3 lbs. fresh Champignons mushrooms
- 1 c. vinegar (for blanching)
- 1 c. water
- 3 chopped garlic cloves
- Sea salt

INGREDIENTS

1. In a saucepan place mushrooms, garlic, salt, water and vinegar.
2. Blanch mushrooms in distilled vinegar bringing to boil.
3. Remove from heat and let cool completely.
4. Store marinated mushrooms in the refrigerator.

NUTRITION VALUES: Calories: 61.51 Fat: 0.79g Carbs: 6.4g Protein: 7.2g

16.   SPICY KALE WITH CHILI FLAKES

Servings: 2

INGREDIENTS

- 3 tbsps. extra-virgin olive oil
- 1 lb. bunch broccoli
- 2 tbsps. water
- 3 smashed garlic cloves
- 1 tsp. crushed red chili flakes
- Kosher salt

DIRECTIONS

1. Heat the oil in a large frying skillet over medium-high heat.
2. Sauté garlic for about 2-3 minutes.
3. Add the broccoli flowerets and sauté, turning occasionally, 6–8 minutes.
4. Sprinkle in 2 tablespoon water and simmer for 2-3 minutes.
5. Add chili flakes and season salt.
6. Cover and cook about 5 minutes.
7. Taste and adjust salt.
8. Serve.

NUTRITION VALUES: Calories: 238.84 Fat: 21g Carbs: 7.21g Protein: 6.36g

SPICY KALE WITH CHILI FLAKES

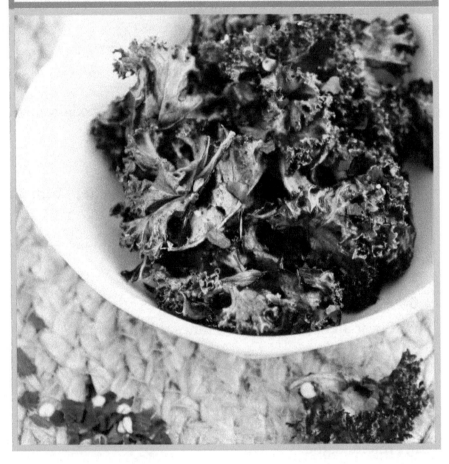

17. SWISH CHARD AND SPINACH WITH FETA

Servings: 4

INGREDIENTS

- ¾ lbs. Swiss chard
- ½ lbs. fresh spinach
- 2 tbsps. Olive oil
- 2 chopped green onions
- 1 bunch of dill
- ¾ lbs. Feta cheese
- Salt
- Black pepper

DIRECTIONS

1. Wash, clean and chop Swish chard and spinach.
2. Heat water with salt in a large pot (3 quart); bring to boil and add chard and spinach to the boiling water. Boil only for 2 -3 minutes.
3. Remove from the water, and drain in a colander.
4. In the same pot, heat the olive oil and sauté onion until soft.
5. Place drained Swish chard and spinach in a pot and stir well.
6. Pour one c. of water and boil for 10-15 minutes; season salt and pepper and add the dill.
7. Let it simmer for 5 minutes until all liquids are absorbed.
8. Add crumbled Feta cheese and slightly stir.

9. Remove from the heat, taste, adjust seasonings and serve.

NUTRITION VALUES: Calories: 315.92 Fat: 25.26g Carbs: 7.29g Protein: 15.38g

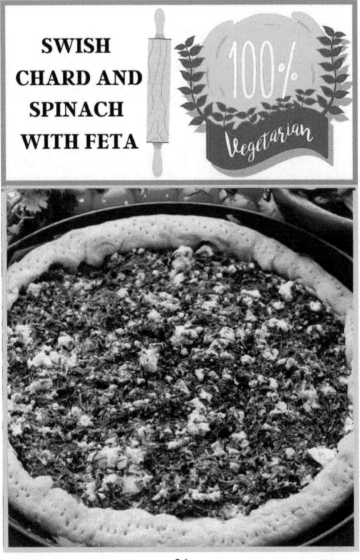

18. <u>WARM SPINACH BASIL SALAD WITH ALMONDS</u>

Servings: 2

INGREDIENTS

- 2 tbsps. Olive oil
- 1 diced green onion
- 1 garlic clove
- 4 c. chopped spinach
- ½ c. basil, fresh
- ½ c. water
- ¼ c. chopped almonds
- Salt
- Pepper

DIRECTIONS

1. Wash and clean your vegetables.
2. Heat the oil in a frying skill over medium heat, and sauté chopped onion and garlic for 3 - 4 minutes.
3. Add spinach, basil, water and salt and pepper. Cover and cook, stirring occasionally, for 5 minutes.
4. Transfer vegetables on a serving plate.
5. Serve warm with chopped almonds.

NUTRITION VALUES: Calories: 242.95 Fat: 22.8g Carbs: 5.19g Protein: 5.92g

19. ARUGULA TOMATO SALAD

Servings: 2

INGREDIENTS

- 4 tbsps. Olive oil
- 1 c. cherry tomatoes
- 3 c. arugula
- 1 chopped red onion
- 4 tbsps. Capers
- 2 tbsps. Chopped basil

DIRECTIONS

1. Add all ingredients into mixing bowl and toss.
2. Serve fresh and enjoy!

NUTRITION VALUES: Calories: 262 Fat: 26.7g Carbs: 6g Protein: 2.1g

Arugula Tomato Salad

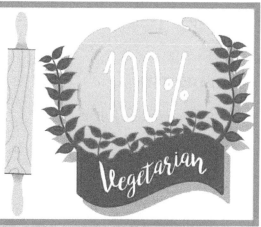

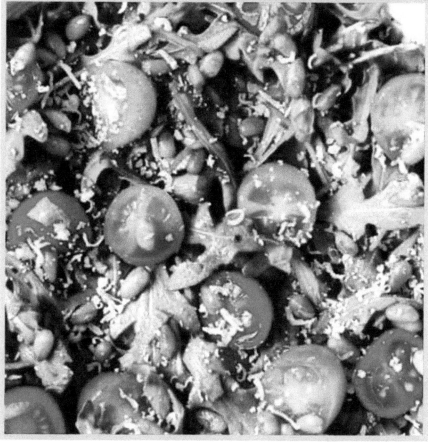

20. SPICY ASIAN BROCCOLI

Servings: 4

INGREDIENTS

- 2 fresh limes' juice
- 2 small broccoli
- 2 tsps. Chopped chili pepper
- 2 tsps. grated ginger
- 4 chopped garlic cloves
- 8 tbsps. olive oil

DIRECTIONS

1. Add your broccoli florets into your steamer and steam them for 8 minutes.
2. Meanwhile, to prepare dressing, add lime juice, garlic, chili pepper, oil, and ginger in a small mixing bowl and combine.
3. Add steamed broccoli in a large mixing bowl and drizzle over it the dressing.
4. Toss to blend.
5. Serve and enjoy!

NUTRITION VALUES: Calories: 294 Fat: 26.6g Carbs: 9.4g Protein: 6.3g

21. DELICIOUS SPANISH CAULIFLOWER RICE

Preparation Time: 20 minutes

Servings: 3

INGREDIENTS

- 1 cauliflower head
- 1/4 cup vegetable broth
- 2 tbsp tomato paste
- 1 tsp cumin
- 3 garlic cloves, minced
- 1/2 cup onion, diced
- 1 tbsp olive oil
- 1 tsp salt

DIRECTIONS

1. Cut the stem of cauliflower and cut cauliflower in half.
2. Add cauliflower in food processor and process until it looks like rice.
3. Heat large pan over medium heat.
4. Add onion to the pan and sauté for 3 minutes.
5. Add minced garlic and sauté for 30 seconds.
6. Add cauliflower rice, cumin, and salt and stir well.
7. Now add tomato paste and broth and stir until tomato paste dissolves completely.
8. Serve hot and enjoy.

NUTRITION VALUES: Calories 89 Fat 5 g Carbohydrates 9 g Sugar 4 g Protein 3 g Cholesterol 0 mg

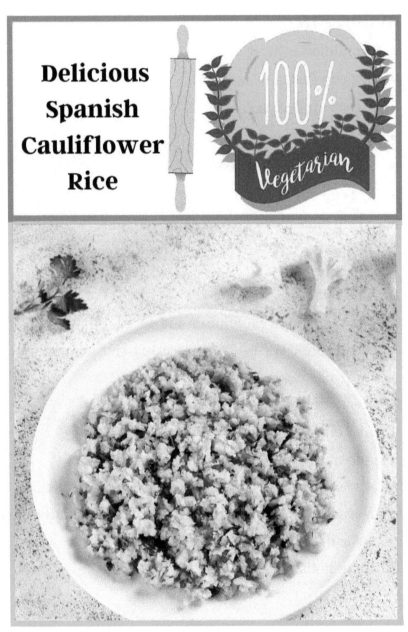

22.   STIR FRIED BROCCOLI

Preparation Time: 20 minutes

Servings: 4

INGREDIENTS

- 1 lb broccoli florets
- 1 tbsp sesame seeds
- 1/2 tsp ground ginger
- 1/3 cup coconut amino
- 2 garlic cloves, minced
- 2 tbsp olive oil
- 1/2 tsp salt

DIRECTIONS

1. Heat oil in a pan over medium-high heat.
2. Add garlic and sauté for 30 seconds.
3. Add broccoli and salt in a pan and sauté for 5 minutes.
4. Combine together ginger and coconut amino.
5. Add coconut amino and ginger mixture in pan and cover pan with a lid.
6. Cook broccoli for some minutes or until softer then removes lid carefully.
7. Remove pan from heat and add sesame seeds and stir well.
8. Serve warm and enjoy.

NUTRITION VALUES: Calories 135 Fat 8 g Carbohydrates 12 g Sugar 2 g

Protein 3 g Cholesterol 0 mg

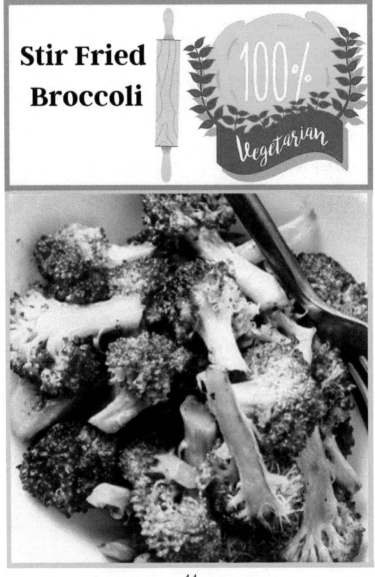

23. TASTY ZUCCHINI GRATIN

Preparation Time: 60 minutes

Servings: 9

INGREDIENTS

- 4 cups raw zucchini, sliced
- 1/2 cup heavy whipping cream
- 1/2 tsp garlic powder
- 2 tbsp butter
- 1 1/2 cups pepper jack cheese, shredded
- 1 onion, sliced
- Pepper
- Salt

DIRECTIONS

1. Preheat the oven to 375 F.
2. Spray oven safe pan with cooking spray.
3. Add 1/3 sliced onion and zucchini in pan and season with pepper and salt.
4. Sprinkle 1/2 cup cheese over sliced onion and zucchini.
5. In a microwave safe dish, combine together heavy whipping cream, butter, and garlic powder.
6. Microwave for 1 minute or until butter is melted.
7. Pour heavy cream mixture over sliced zucchini and onion.

8. Bake in preheated oven for 45 minutes or until top lightly golden brown.

9. Serve warm and enjoy.

NUTRITION VALUES: Calories 87 Fat 6 g Carbohydrates 3 g Sugar 1 g Protein 1 g Cholesterol 18 mg

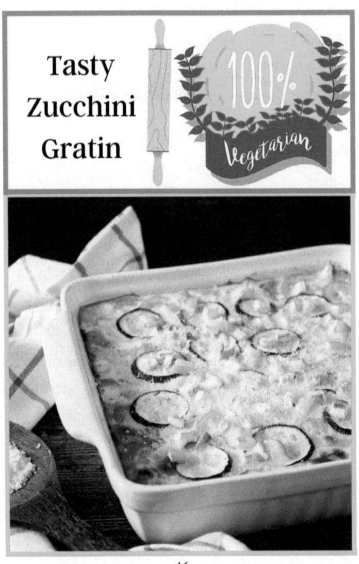

Tasty Zucchini Gratin

100%

Vegetarian

24.   ZUCCHINI CHEESE NOODLES

Preparation Time: 20 minutes

Servings: 2

INGREDIENTS

- 1 zucchini
- 2/3 cup cheddar cheese, shredded
- 2 tbsp almond milk
- 1 tbsp butter
- 1/2 cup water
- 1 tsp salt

DIRECTIONS

1. Cut the ends of zucchini and using spiralizer make zucchini noodles.
2. Add noodles, salt, and water in a saucepan and bring to boil. Boil noodles until soft and water are completely absorbed.
3. Reduce heat to low and add cheese, almond milk, and butter.
4. Stir well to combine.
5. Serve hot and enjoy.

NUTRITION VALUES: Calories 253 Fat 22 g Carbohydrates 4 g Sugar 2 g Protein 11 g Cholesterol 55 mg

Zucchini Cheese Noodles

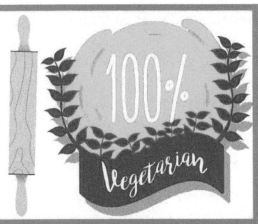

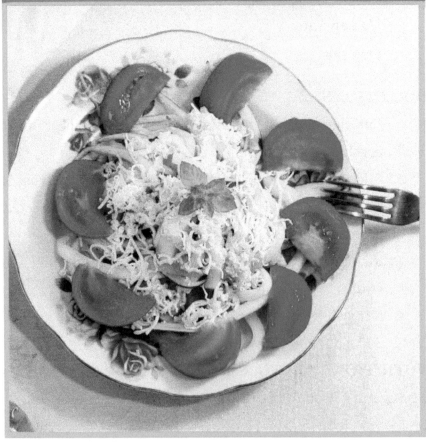

25. MUSHROOM SPINACH QUICHE

Preparation Time: 55 minutes

Servings: 6

INGREDIENTS

- 8 oz mushrooms, sliced
- 10 oz frozen spinach, thawed
- 1/2 cup mozzarella cheese, shredded
- 1/4 cup parmesan cheese, grated
- 2 oz feta cheese, crumbled
- 1 cup almond milk
- 4 large eggs
- 1 garlic clove, minced
- Pepper
- Salt

DIRECTIONS

1. Preheat the oven to 350 F.
2. Spray pan with cooking spray and heat over medium heat.
3. Add garlic, mushrooms, pepper and salt in a pan and sauté for 5 minutes.
4. Spray a 9-inch pie dish with cooking spray.
5. Place spinach in the bottom of dish then places sautéed mushroom over spinach.

6. Sprinkle crumbled feta cheese over spinach and mushroom layer.

7. In a bowl, whisk together eggs, parmesan cheese, and almond milk.

8. Pour egg mixture over spinach and mushroom layer then sprinkle shredded mozzarella cheese.

9. Bake in preheated oven for 45 minutes or until lightly golden brown.

10. Cut quiche into slices and serve.

NUTRITION VALUES: Calories 221 Fat 17 g Carbohydrates 6 g Sugar 2 g Protein 12 g Cholesterol 140 mg

Mushroom Spinach Quiche

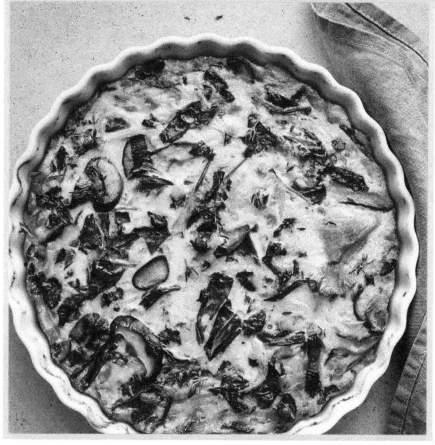

26. DELICIOUS EGGPLANT GRATIN

Preparation Time: 40 minutes

Servings: 6

INGREDIENTS

- 2 lbs eggplant, cut into 1/2 inch slices
- 3/4 cup heavy whipping cream
- 6 tbsp cheese, shredded
- 6 tbsp fresh parsley, chopped
- 1 tbsp mint, dried
- 1/3 lb feta cheese, crumbled
- 2 tbsp olive oil
- 2 onions, sliced
- Pepper
- Salt

DIRECTIONS

1. Brush olive oil on both sides of sliced eggplants and place in baking tray.
2. Season sliced eggplants with salt and bake at 400 F until lightly golden brown.
3. Meanwhile, heat little oil in a pan over medium heat.
4. Add sliced onion to the pan and sauté until lightly brown.
5. Place fried onion over baked eggplants then add parsley and mint.
6. Now top with grated cheese and feta cheese.

7. Pour heavy whipped cream over eggplant and onion layer.

8. Bake at 450 F for 30 minutes or gratin lightly brown.

9. Serve and enjoy.

NUTRITION VALUES: Calories 241 Fat 18 g Carbohydrates 13 g Sugar 7 g Protein 7 g Cholesterol 50 mg

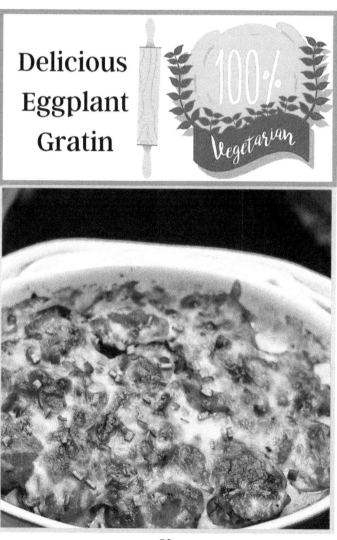

27.   AVOCADO CHEESE TOMATO SALAD

Preparation Time: 15 minutes

Servings: 3

INGREDIENTS

- 4 medium tomatoes, sliced
- 2 tbsp olive oil
- 2 tbsp pesto
- 4 oz mozzarella cheese
- 6 kalamata olives, halved and deseed
- 1 large avocado, peel and sliced
- Pepper
- Salt

DIRECTIONS

1. Add avocado, olives, and tomato in a bowl and mix well.
2. Add olive oil, pesto, and mozzarella.
3. Season with pepper and salt.
4. Toss well and serve.

NUTRITION VALUES: Calories 408 Fat 34 g Carbohydrates 13 g Sugar 5 g Protein 14 g Cholesterol 23 mg

28.   CLASSIC GREEK SALAD

Preparation Time: 15 minutes

Servings: 4

INGREDIENTS

- 4 medium tomatoes, sliced
- 4 tbsp olive oil
- 1 tsp oregano, dried
- 7 oz feta cheese, crumbled
- 4 tbsp capers
- 16 kalamata olives
- 1 small onion, sliced
- 1 medium green pepper, sliced
- 1 large cucumber, peel and sliced
- Pepper
- Salt

DIRECTIONS

1. Add all ingredients to the bowl and toss well.
2. Serve immediately and enjoy.

NUTRITION VALUES: Calories 321 Fat 27 g Carbohydrates 14 g Sugar 8 g Protein 9 g Cholesterol 44 mg

Classic Greek Salad

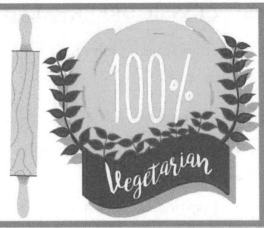

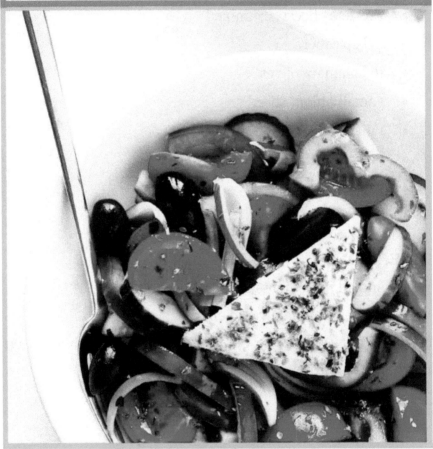

29.   TOFU PESTO ZOODLES

Preparation Time: 5 minutes

Cooking Time: 12 minutes

Servings: 4

INGREDIENTS

- 2 tbsp olive oil
- 1 medium white onion, chopped
- 1 garlic clove, minced
- 2 (14 oz) blocks firm tofu, soaked and cubed
- 1 medium red bell pepper, deseeded and sliced
- 6 medium zucchinis, spiralized
- ¼ cup basil pesto, olive oil-based
- Salt and freshly ground black pepper to taste
- ½ cup shredded Gouda cheese
- 2/3 cup grated Parmesan cheese
- Toasted pine nuts to garnish

DIRECTIONS

1. Over medium fire, heat olive oil in a medium pot and sauté onion and garlic until softened and fragrant, 3 minutes.
2. Add tofu and cook until golden on all sides. Pour in bell pepper and cook until softened, 4 minutes.
3. Mix in zucchinis, pesto, salt, and black pepper. Cook for 3 minutes or until zucchinis soften slightly. Turn heat off and carefully mix in Gouda cheese to melt.

4. Dish into four plates, top with Parmesan cheese, pine nuts, and serve.

NUTRITION VALUES: Calories 477, Total Fat 32g, Total Carbs 12.04, Fiber 6.6g, Net Carbs 5.44g, Protein 20.42

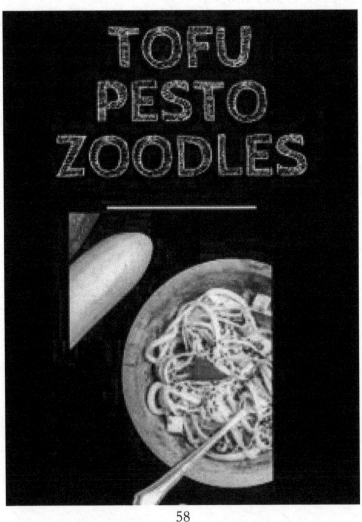

30. <u>CHEESY MUSHROOM PIE</u>

Preparation Time: 10 minutes

Cooking Time: 43 minutes + 1 hour refrigeration

Servings: 4

INGREDIENTS

For piecrust:

- 3 tbsp coconut flour
- ¼ cup almond flour + extra for dusting
- ½ tsp salt
- ¼ cup butter, cold and crumbled
- 3 tbsp swerve sugar
- 1 ½ tsp vanilla extract
- 4 whole eggs, cracked into a bowl

For filling:

- 2 tbsp butter
- 1 medium brown onion
- 2 garlic cloves, minced
- 1 green bell pepper, deseeded and diced
- 1 cup green beans, cut into 3 pieces each
- 2 cups mixed mushrooms, chopped
- Salt and freshly ground black pepper to taste
- ¼ cup coconut cream
- 1/3 cup sour cream
- ½ cup unsweetened almond milk
- 2 eggs, lightly beaten

- ¼ tsp nutmeg powder
- 1 tbsp freshly chopped parsley
- 1 cup grated cheddar cheese

DIRECTIONS

For piecrust:

1. Preheat oven to 350∘F and grease a pie pan with cooking spray. Set aside.
2. In a large bowl, combine coconut flour, almond flour, and salt.
3. Add butter and mix with an electric hand mixer until crumbly. Add swerve sugar, vanilla extract, and mix well. Pour in eggs one after another while mixing until formed into a ball.
4. Flatten dough on a chopping board, cover in plastic wrap, and refrigerate for 1 hour.
5. Lightly dust chopping board with almond flour, unwrap dough, and roll out into a large rectangle of ½-inch thickness. Fit dough in pie pan, and cover with parchment paper.
6. Pour in some baking beans and bake in oven until golden, 10 minutes. Remove after, pour out beans, remove parchment paper, and allow cooling.

For filling:

1. Meanwhile, melt butter in a skillet and sauté onion and garlic until softened and fragrant, 3 minutes. Add bell

pepper, green beans, mushroom, salt and black pepper; cook for 5 minutes.

2. In a medium bowl, beat coconut cream, sour cream, almond milk, and eggs. Season with salt, black pepper, and nutmeg. Stir in parsley and cheddar cheese.

3. Spread mushroom mixture in baked crust and top with cheese filling.

4. Bake until golden on top and cheese melted, 20 to 25 minutes.

5. Remove; allow cooling for 10 minutes, slice, and serve.

NUTRITION VALUES: Calories 527, Total Fat 43.58g, Total Carbs 8.73g, Fiber 2.2g, Net Carbs 6.53g, Protein 21.3g

31. <u>__MEATLESS FLORENTINE PIZZA__</u>

Preparation Time: 10 minutes

Cooking Time: 25 minutes

Servings: 2

INGREDIENTS

For pizza crust:

- 6 eggs
- 1 tsp Italian seasoning
- 1 cup shredded provolone cheese

For topping:

- 2/3 cup tomato sauce
- 2 cups baby spinach, wilted
- ½ cup grated mozzarella cheese
- 1 (7 oz) can sliced mushrooms, drained
- 4 eggs
- Olive oil for drizzling

DIRECTIONS

For pizza crust:

1. Preheat oven to 400° F and line a pizza pan with parchment paper. Set aside.
2. Crack eggs into a medium bowl and whisk in Italian seasoning and provolone cheese.
3. Spread mixture on pizza pan and bake until golden, 10 minutes. Remove and allow cooling for 2 minutes.

For pizza:

1. Increase oven's temperature to 450° F.
2. Spread tomato sauce on crust, top with spinach, mozzarella cheese, and mushrooms. Bake for 8 minutes.
3. Crack eggs on top and continue baking until eggs set, 2 minutes.
4. Remove, slice, and serve.

NUTRITION VALUES: Calories 646, Total Fat 39.19g, Total Carbs 8.42g, Fiber 3.5g, Net Carbs 4.92g, Protein 36.87g

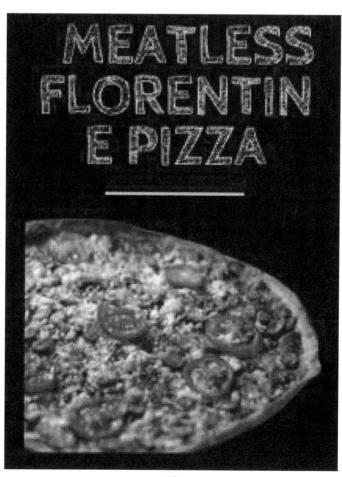

32. MARGHERITA PIZZA WITH CAULIFLOWER CRUST

Preparation Time: 8 minutes

Cooking Time: 30 minutes

Servings: 2

INGREDIENTS

For pizza crust:

- 2 cups cauliflower rice
- 4 eggs
- ¼ cup shredded Monterey Jack cheese
- ¼ cup shredded Parmesan cheese
- ½ tsp Italian seasoning
- Salt and freshly ground black pepper to taste

For topping:

- 6 tbsp unsweetened tomato sauce
- 1 small red onion, thinly sliced
- 2 ½ oz cremini mushrooms, sliced
- 1 tsp dried oregano
- ½ cup cottage cheese
- ½ tbsp. olive oil
- A handful fresh basil

DIRECTIONS

For pizza crust:

1. Preheat oven to 400° F and line a baking sheet with parchment paper.

2. Pour cauliflower into a safe microwave bowl, sprinkle with 1 tablespoon of water, cover with plastic wrap and microwave for 1 to 2 minutes or until softened. Remove and allow cooling.

3. Pour cauliflower into a cheesecloth and squeeze out as much liquid. Transfer to a mixing bowl.

4. Crack in eggs, add cheeses, Italian seasoning, salt, and black pepper. Mix until well-combined.

5. Spread mixture on baking sheet and bake in oven until golden, 15 minutes.

6. Remove from oven and allow cooling for 2 minutes.

For topping:

1. Spread tomato sauce on pizza crust, scatter onion and mushrooms on top, sprinkle with oregano, and add cottage cheese. Drizzle with olive oil and bake until golden, 15 minutes.

2. Remove, top with basil, slice and serve.

NUTRITION VALUES: Calories 290, Total Fat 22.58g, Total Carbs 6.62g, Fiber 5.8g, Net Carbs 0.82g, Protein 12.81g

MARGHERITA PIZZA WITH CAULIFLOWER CRUST

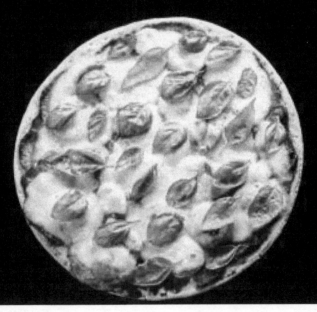

33. ALMOND TOFU LOAF

Preparation Time: 10 minutes

Cooking Time: 1 hour

Servings: 4

INGREDIENTS

- 3 tbsp olive oil + extra for brushing
- 4 garlic cloves, minced
- 2 white onions, finely chopped
- 1 lb firm tofu, pressed and cubed
- 2 tbsp coconut aminos
- ¾ cup chopped almonds
- Salt and freshly ground black pepper
- 1 tbsp dried mixed herbs
- ½ tsp erythritol
- ¼ cup golden flax seed meal
- 1 tbsp sesame seeds
- 1 cup chopped mixed bell peppers
- ½ cup tomato sauce

DIRECTIONS

1. Preheat oven to 350°F and lightly brush an 8 x 4 inch loaf pan with olive oil. Set aside.
2. In a medium bowl, combine olive oil, garlic, onion, tofu, coconut aminos, almonds, salt, black pepper, mixed herbs, erythritol, golden flax seed meal, sesame seeds, and bell peppers, and mix well.

3. Fit mixture in loaf pan, spread tomato sauce on top, and bake in oven for 45 minutes to 1 hour.

4. Remove pan and turn tofu loaf over onto a chopping board.

5. Slice and serve with garden green salad.

NUTRITION VALUES: Calories 432, Total Fat 31.38g, Total Carbs 8.74g, Fiber 6.2g, Net Carbs 2.54g, Protein 24.36g

34. KALE AND MUSHROOM BIRYANI

Preparation Time: 15 minutes

Cooking Time: 46 minutes

Servings: 4

INGREDIENTS

- 6 cups cauli rice
- 2 tbsp water
- Salt and freshly ground black pepper
- 3 tbsp ghee
- 3 medium white onions, chopped
- 1 tsp ginger puree
- 1 tbsp turmeric powder + more for dusting
- 2 cups chopped tomatoes
- 1 red chili, finely chopped
- 1 tbsp tomato puree
- 1 cup sliced cremini mushrooms
- 1 cup diced paneer cheese
- 1 cup kale, chopped
- 1/3 cup water
- 1 cup plain yogurt
- ¼ cup chopped cilantro
- Olive oil for drizzling

DIRECTIONS

1. Preheat oven to 400° F.

2. Pour cauliflower rice into a safe microwave bowl, drizzle with water, cover with plastic wrap, and microwave for 1 minute or until softened. Remove and season with salt and black pepper. Set aside.

3. Melt ghee in a casserole pan and sauté onion, ginger, and turmeric powder. Cook until fragrant, 5 minutes.

4. Add tomatoes, red chili, and tomato puree; cook until tomatoes soften, 5 minutes.

5. Stir in mushrooms, paneer cheese, kale, and water; season with salt and black pepper and simmer until mushrooms soften, 10 minutes. Turn heat off and stir in yogurt.

6. Spoon half of stew into a bowl and set aside. Sprinkle half of cilantro on remaining stew in casserole pan, top with half of cauli rice, and dust with turmeric. Repeat layering a second time with remaining ingredients.

7. Drizzle with olive oil and bake until golden and crisp on top, 25 minutes.

8. Remove; allow cooling, and serve with coconut chutney.

NUTRITION VALUES: Calories 346, Total Fat 21.48g, Total Carbs 8.63g, Fiber 6.6g, Net Carbs 2.03g, Protein 16.01g

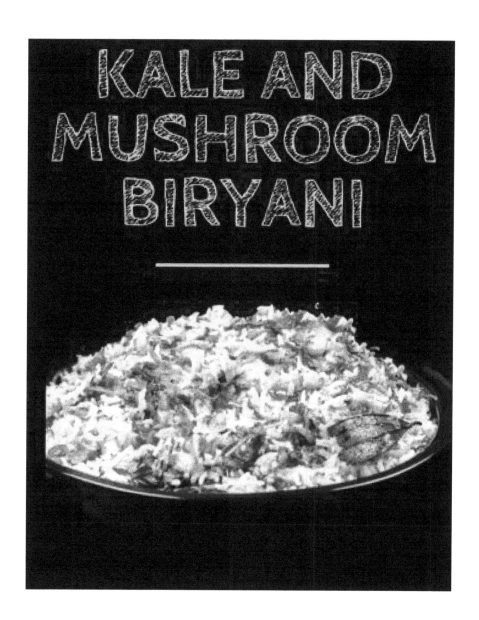

KALE AND MUSHROOM BIRYANI

35. <u>MUSHROOM PIZZA BOWLS WITH AVOCADO & CILANTRO</u>

Preparation Time: 15 minutes

Cooking Time: 17 minutes

Servings: 4

INGREDIENTS

- 1 ½ cups broccoli rice
- 2 tbsp water
- Olive oil for brushing
- 2 cups unsweetened pizza sauce
- 1 cup grated Gruyere cheese
- 1 cup grated mozzarella cheese
- 2 large tomatoes, chopped
- ½ cup sliced cremini mushrooms
- 1 small red onion, chopped
- 1 tsp dried basil
- Salt and freshly ground black pepper to taste
- 1 avocado, halved, pitted, and chopped
- ¼ cup chopped parsley

DIRECTIONS

1. Preheat oven to 400° F.
2. Pour broccoli rice into a safe microwave bowl, drizzle with water, and steam in microwave for 1 to 2 minutes. Remove, fluff with a fork, and set aside.

3. Lightly brush the inner parts of four medium ramekins with olive oil and spread in half of pizza sauce. Top with half of broccoli rice and half of cheeses.

4. In a bowl, combine tomatoes, mushrooms, onion, basil, salt, and black pepper. Spoon half of mixture into ramekins and top with half of cheeses. Repeat layering a second time making sure to finish off with cheeses.

5. Bake until cheese melts and golden on top, 15 minutes.

6. Remove ramekins and top with avocados and parsley.

7. Allow cooling for 3 minutes and serve.

NUTRITION VALUES: Calories 378, Total Fat 22.54g, Total Carbs 12.27g, Fiber 8.9g, Net Carbs 3.37g, Protein 20.68g

36. PISTACHIOS AND CHEESE STUFFED ZUCCHINIS

Preparation Time: 15 minutes

Cooking Time: 17 minutes

Servings: 4

INGREDIENTS

- 1 cup riced broccoli
- ¼ cup vegetable broth
- 4 medium zucchinis, halved
- 2 tbsp olive oil + more for drizzling
- 1 ¼ cup diced tomatoes
- 1 medium red onion, chopped
- ¼ cup pine nuts
- ¼ cup chopped pistachios
- 4 tbsp chopped parsley
- 1 tbsp smoked paprika
- 1 tbsp balsamic vinegar
- Salt and freshly ground black pepper to taste
- 1 cup grated Parmesan cheese

DIRECTIONS

1. Preheat oven to 350°F.
2. Pour broccoli rice and vegetable broth in a medium pot and cook over medium heat until softened, 2 minutes. Turn heat off, fluff broccoli rice, and allow cooling.

3. Scoop flesh out of zucchini halves, chop pulp and set aside. Brush zucchini boats with some olive oil. Set aside.

4. In a medium bowl, combine broccoli rice, tomatoes, red onion, pine nuts, pistachios, parsley, paprika, balsamic vinegar, zucchini pulp, salt, and black pepper.

5. Spoon mixture into zucchini boats, drizzle with more olive oil, and cover top with Parmesan cheese.

6. Place filled zucchinis on a baking sheet and bake until cheese melts and is golden, 15 minutes.

7. Remove, allow cooling, and serve.

NUTRITION VALUES: Calories 330, Total Fat 28.12g, Total Carbs 10.62g, Fiber 5.4g, Net Carbs 5.22g, Protein 12.3g

37. <u>SOY CHORIZO-ASPARAGUS BOWL</u>

Preparation Time: 15 minutes

Cooking Time: 15 minutes

Servings: 4

INGREDIENTS

- 1 lb soy chorizo, cubed
- 1 lb asparagus, trimmed and halved
- 1 cup green beans, trimmed
- 1 cup chopped mixed bell peppers
- 2 red onions, cut into wedges
- 1 head medium broccoli, cut into florets
- 2 rosemary sprigs
- Salt and freshly ground black pepper to taste
- 4 tbsp olive oil
- 1 tbsp maple (sugar-free) syrup
- 1 lemon, juiced

DIRECTIONS

1. Preheat oven to 400° F.
2. On a baking tray, spread soy chorizo, asparagus, green beans, bell peppers, onions, broccoli, and rosemary. Season with salt, black pepper, and drizzle with olive oil and maple syrup. Rub spices into vegetables.
3. Bake until vegetables soften and light brown around the edges, 15 minutes.

4. Dish vegetables into serving bowls, drizzle with lemon juice, and serve warm.

NUTRITION VALUES: Calories 300, Total Fat 18.55g, Total Carbs 12.5g, Fiber 9.2g, Net Carbs 3.3g, Protein 14.87g

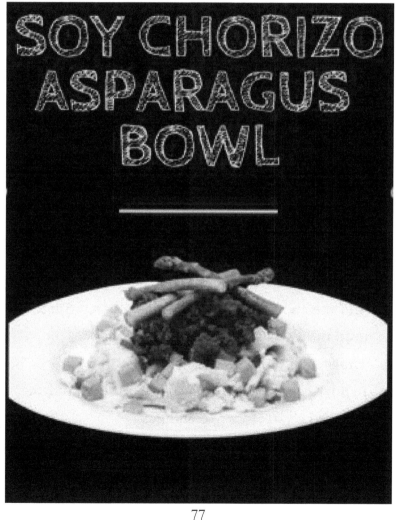

38. ANTIOXIDANT ZUCCHINI, LETTUCE AND RADICCHIO SALAD

Servings: 4

INGREDIENTS

- 4 boiled zucchini
- 1 large lettuce head
- 2 chopped celery stalk
- ½ c. chopped almonds
- 4 sliced radishes,
- Olive oil (extra virgin)
- 1 lemon juice
- 4 tbsps. Parmesan cheese
- Salt
- Pepper

DIRECTIONS

1. Wash and slice your zucchini.
2. Heat the water in a pot over the medium heat.
3. Add the zucchini, cover and cook for 3 to 6 minutes or until the squash is tender.
4. Transfer zucchini in colander and drain well.
5. In a large bowl place lettuce, celery, sliced radishes and chopped celery; toss to combine.
6. Pour olive oil, lemon juice and sprinkle with Parmesan cheese; toss.

7. Serve.

NUTRITION VALUES: Calories: 168.4 Fat: 11.16g Carbs: 6.45g Protein: 8.4g

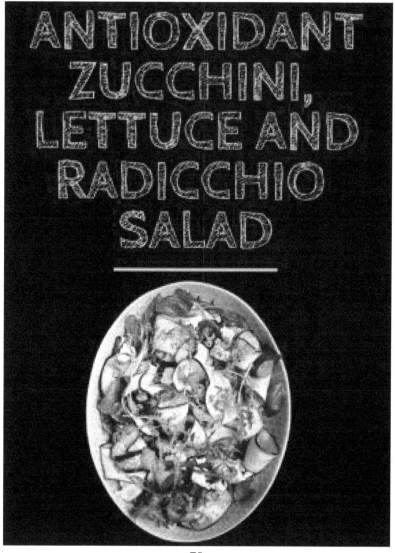

39. BAKED PUMPKIN "SPAGHETTI" WITH HERBES DE PROVENCE

Servings: 6

INGREDIENTS

- 1 large pumpkin for spaghetti squash
- ½ c. grass-fed butter
- 3 tsps. Herbes de Provence
- 1 pressed garlic clove
- 1 chopped scallion
- 1 tsp. lemon juice
- 4 tbsps. Grated Parmesan
- Salt
- Black pepper

DIRECTIONS

1. Preheat the oven to 375F.
2. Wash the pumpkin and cut in half.
3. In a shallow baking dish, add two halves face down and cover with foil.
4. Bake for 1 - 1 1/2 hours.
5. Mix the butter with the herbs, onion, pressed garlic and the lemon juice until creamy.
6. When the pumpkin is cooked, remove the seeds and remove the pulp with a fork (this produces wonderful spaghetti-like threads.

7. Place the pumpkin "spaghetti" and season with salt and pepper to taste.
8. Pour with the butter/herb mixture, sprinkle with the Parmesan and serve immediately.

NUTRITION VALUES: Calories: 204.22 Fat: 17.72g Carbs: 7.17g Protein: 3.7g

40. CABBAGE, CAULIFLOWER, AND LEEK PUREE

Servings: 4

INGREDIENTS

- ½ medium cabbage head
- 1 leek
- 4 c. cauliflower florets
- 2 tbsps. Olive oil
- Chopped Parsley
- Salt
- Pepper

DIRECTIONS

1. Chop the vegetables and wash well.
2. Heat water in a big pot and place the vegetables; season with salt.
3. Bring to boil, reduce the heat, cover and cook it 15 -20 minutes, until the vegetables are soft.
4. Transfer vegetables in a blender or food processor and add the oil; blend until smooth.
5. Taste and adjust salt and pepper.
6. Decorate with chopped parsley (optional) and serve.

NUTRITION VALUES: Calories: 128.37 Fat: 7.23g Carbs: 7.05g Protein: 3.84g

41. <u>CHILLED AVOCADO AND ENDIVE SOUP</u>

Servings: 3

INGREDIENTS

- 3 endives
- 2 chopped spring onions
- 1 diced avocado
- 1 c. Greek yogurt
- 1 tbsp. olive oil
- 1 chopped garlic clove
- 3 cardamom seeds
- 4 chopped mint leaves
- Salt

DIRECTIONS

1. Place all ingredients from the list in your high speed blender.
2. Blend until smooth and creamy.
3. Refrigerate for 2-3 hours and serve cold.

NUTRITION VALUES: Calories: 193.1 Fat: 14.69g Carbs: 7.99g Protein: 5.71g

CHILLED AVOCADO AND ENDIVE SOUP

42. CREAMY WATERCRESS LUNCH DIP

Servings: 2

INGREDIENTS

- ½ lb. watercress
- 1½ c. cottage cheese
- ¾ c. Mayonnaise (gluten-free, grain free)
- ½ c. chopped chives and parsley
- 3 tbsps. Lemon juice
- Kosher salt
- Black pepper

DIRECTIONS

1. Place all ingredients from the list (watercress, cottage cheese, Mayonnaise (gluten-free, grain free), chives and parsley, lemon juice and salt) in your fast-speed blender.
2. Blend on HIGH speed until smooth.
3. Refrigerate for 1-2 hours.
4. Serve.

NUTRITION VALUES: Calories:31963 Fat: 17.49g Carbs 9.13g Protein: 23.49g

CREAMY WATERCRESS LUNCH DIP

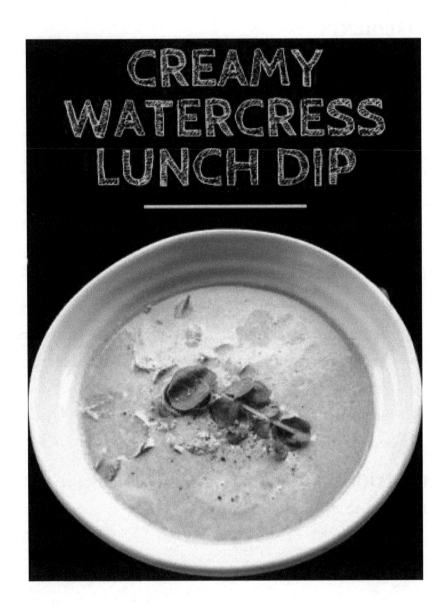

SIDES

43. SOY CHORIZO STUFFED CABBAGE ROLLS

Preparation Time: 5 minutes

Cooking Time: 30 minutes

Servings: 4

INGREDIENTS

- ¼ cup coconut oil, divided
- 1 large white onion, chopped, divided
- 3 cloves garlic, minced, divided
- 1 cup crumbled soy chorizo
- 1 cup cauliflower rice
- Salt and freshly ground black pepper to taste
- 1 can tomato sauce
- 1 tsp dried oregano
- 1 tsp dried basil
- ¼ cup water
- 8 full green cabbage leaves

DIRECTIONS

1. Heat half of the coconut oil in a saucepan over medium heat.

2. Add half of the onion, half of the garlic, and all of the soy chorizo. Sauté for 5 minutes or until the chorizo has browned further and the onion softened.

3. Stir in the cauli rice, season with salt and black pepper, and cook for 3 to 4 minutes. Turn the heat off and set the pot aside.

4. Heat the remaining oil in a saucepan over medium heat, add, and sauté the remaining onion and garlic until fragrant and soft.

5. Pour in the tomato sauce, and season with salt, black pepper, oregano, and basil. Add the water and simmer the sauce for 10 minutes.

6. While the sauce cooks, lay the cabbage leaves on a flat surface, and spoon the soy chorizo mixture into the middle of each leaf. Roll the leaves to secure the filling.

7. Place the cabbage rolls in the tomato sauce and cook further for 10 minutes.

8. When ready, serve the cabbage rolls with sauce over mashed broccoli or with mixed seed bread.

NUTRITION VALUES: Calories: 285; Total Fat: 26g; Total Carbs: 7g; Fiber: 5g; Net Carbs: 7g; Protein: 5g

44. ONION RINGS AND KALE DIP

Preparation Time: 15 minutes

Cooking Time: 20 minutes

Servings: 4

INGREDIENTS
Onion Rings:

- 1 large white onion
- 1 tbsp flax seed meal + 3 tbsp water
- 1 cup almond flour
- ½ cup grated vegan parmesan
- 1 tsp garlic powder
- ½ tbsp sweet paprika powder
- 1 pinch salt
- Non-stick cooking spray

Kale Dip:

- 2 oz. frozen chopped kale
- 2 tbsp olive oil
- 2 tbsp dried cilantro
- 1 tbsp dried oregano
- 1 tsp garlic powder
- ½ tsp salt
- ¼ tsp freshly ground black pepper
- 1 cup vegan mayonnaise
- 4 tbsp coconut cream

- Juice of ½ a lemon

DIRECTIONS

For the onion rings:

1. Preheat the oven to 400 F.

2. Peel the onion and slice into 1-inch rings. Separate the rings.

3. In a small bowl, mix the flax seed meal and water and leave the mixture to thicken and fully absorb for 5 minutes.

4. Then, in another bowl, combine the almond flour, vegan parmesan, garlic powder, sweet paprika, and salt.

5. Line a baking sheet with parchment paper in readiness for the rings.

6. When the flax egg is ready, dip in the onion rings one after another, and then into the almond flour mixture.

7. Place the rings on the baking sheet and oil with cooking spray.

8. Bake in the oven for 15 to 20 minutes or until golden brown and crispy.

9. Remove the onion rings into a serving bowl.

For the kale dip:

1. While the onion rings crisp, quickly make the dip.

2. Thaw the chopped kale, squeeze out any excess liquid and put in a bowl. Add the olive oil, cilantro, oregano,

garlic powder, salt, black pepper, vegan mayonnaise, coconut cream, and lemon juice. Mix the ingredients until nice and smooth.

3. Allow the dip to sit for about 10 minutes for the flavors to develop. After, serve the dip with the crispy onion rings.

NUTRITION VALUES: Calories: 410; Total Fat: 35g; Total Carbs: 10g; Fiber: 3g; Net Carbs: 7g; Protein: 14g

45. **CURRY CAULI RICE WITH MUSHROOMS**

Preparation Time: 5 minutes

Cooking Time: 10 minutes

Servings: 4

INGREDIENTS

- 2 large heads cauliflower, leaves removed
- 2 tbsp toasted sesame oil, divided
- 1 onion, chopped
- 8 oz baby bella mushrooms, stemmed and sliced
- 3 garlic cloves, minced
- ½ tsp salt
- ¼ tsp freshly ground black pepper
- ½ tsp curry powder
- 1 tsp freshly chopped parsley
- 2 scallions, thinly sliced

DIRECTIONS

1. Use a knife to cut the entire cauliflower head into 6 pieces and transfer to a food processor. With the grater attachment, shred the cauliflower into a rice-like consistency.

2. Heat half of the sesame oil in a large skillet over medium heat, and then add the onion and mushrooms. Sauté for 5 minutes or until the mushrooms are soft.

3. Add the garlic and sauté for 2 minutes or until fragrant. Pour in the cauliflower and cook until the rice has slightly softened about 10 minutes.

4. Season with salt, black pepper, and curry powder; then, mix the ingredients to be well combined. After, turn the heat off and stir in the parsley and scallions. Dish the cauli rice into serving plates and serve warm as a compliment for salads, barbecues, and soups.

NUTRITION VALUES: Calories: 305; Total Fat: 25g; Total Carbs: 14g; Fiber: 5g; Net Carbs: 7g; Protein: 6g

46. MUSHROOM BROCCOLI FAUX RISOTTO

Preparation Time: 5 minutes

Cooking Time: 18 minutes

Servings: 4

INGREDIENTS

- 4 oz. vegan butter
- 1 cup cremini mushrooms, chopped
- 2 garlic cloves, minced
- 1 small red onion, finely chopped
- 1 large head broccoli, coarsely grated
- 1 cup water
- ¾ cup white wine
- Salt and black pepper to taste
- 1 cup coconut whipping cream
- ¾ cup coarsely grated vegan parmesan
- Freshly chopped thyme

DIRECTIONS

1. Place a pot over medium heat, add, and melt the vegan butter. Sauté the mushrooms in the pot until golden, about 5 minutes. Add the garlic and onions and cook for 3 minutes or until fragrant and soft. Mix in the broccoli, water, and half of the white wine. Season with salt and black pepper and simmer the ingredients (uncovered) for 8 to 10 minutes or until the broccoli is soft.

2. Mix in the coconut whipping cream and simmer until most of the cream has evaporated. Turn the heat off and stir in the parmesan cheese and thyme until well incorporated. Dish the risotto and serve warm as itself or with grilled tofu.

NUTRITION VALUES: Calories: 520; Total Fat: 43g; Total Carbs: 18g; Fiber: 6g; Net Carbs: 12g; Protein: 15g

Mushroom Broccoli Faux Risotto

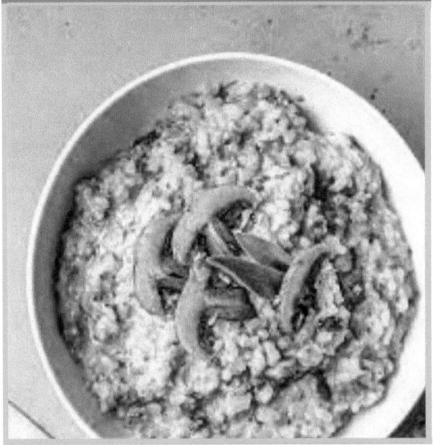

47. __CRISPY SQUASH NACHO CHIPS__

Preparation Time: 6 minutes

Cooking Time: 20 minutes

Servings: 4

INGREDIENTS

- 1 large yellow squash
- Salt to season
- 1 ½ cups coconut oil
- 1 tbsp taco seasoning

DIRECTIONS

1. With a mandolin slicer, cut the squash into thin, round slices and place in a colander.

2. Sprinkle the squash with a lot of salt and allow sitting for 5 minutes. After, press the water out of the squash and pat dry with a paper towel. Pour the coconut oil in a deep skillet and heat the oil over medium heat.

3. Carefully, add the squash slices in the oil, about 20 pieces at a time and fry until crispy and golden brown. Use a slotted spoon to remove the squash onto a paper towel-lined plate. Sprinkle the slices with taco seasoning and serve.

NUTRITION VALUES: Calories: 150; Total Fat: 14g; Total Carbs: 3g; Fiber: 2g; Net Carbs: 1g; Protein: 2g

Crispy Squash Nacho Chips

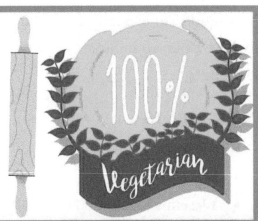

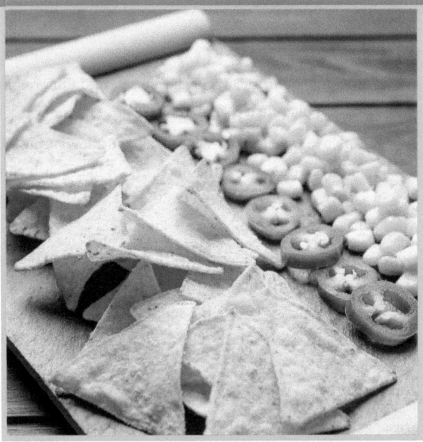

48. <u>TOFU STUFFED PEPPERS</u>

Preparation Time: 5 minutes

Cooking Time: 20 minutes

Servings: 4

INGREDIENTS

- 1 cup mini red and yellow bell peppers
- 1 oz. tofu, chopped into small bits
- 1 tbsp fresh parsley, chopped
- 1 cup dairy - free cream cheese
- ½ - 1 tbsp chili paste, mild
- 2 tbsp melted vegan butter
- Cooking spray
- 1 cup shredded vegan parmesan

DIRECTIONS

1. Preheat the oven to 400 F. Use a knife to cut the bell peppers into two (lengthwise) and remove the core.

2. In a bowl, mix the tofu with parsley, cream cheese, chili paste, and melted butter until smooth.

3. Spoon the cheese mixture into the bell peppers and use the back of the spoon to level the filling in the peppers. Grease a baking sheet with cooking spray and arrange the stuffed peppers on the sheet.

4. Sprinkle the vegan parmesan on top and bake the peppers for 15 to 20 minutes until the peppers are golden

brown and the cheese melted. Remove onto a serving platter and serve warm.

NUTRITION VALUES: Calories: 412; Total Fat: 36g; Total Carbs: 8g; Fiber: 3g; Net Carbs: 5g; Protein: 14g

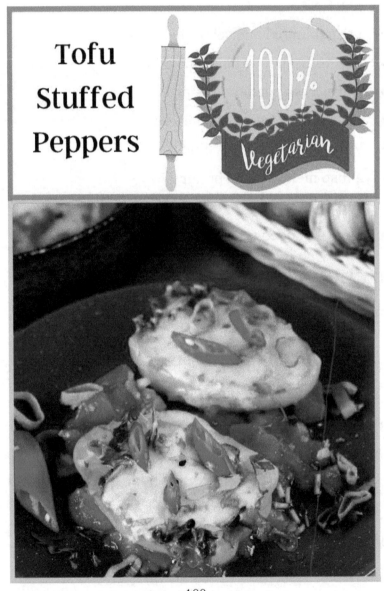

49. MIXED SEED CRACKERS

Preparation Time: 12 minutes

Cooking Time: 45 minutes

Servings: 6

INGREDIENTS

- ⅓ cup sesame seed flour
- ⅓ cup pumpkin seeds
- ⅓ cup sunflower seeds
- ⅓ cup sesame seeds
- ⅓ cup chia seeds
- 1 tbsp psyllium husk powder
- 1 tsp salt
- ¼ cup vegan butter, melted
- 1 cup boiling water

DIRECTIONS

1. Preheat the oven to 300 F.

2. Combine the sesame seed flour with the pumpkin seeds, sunflower seeds, sesame seeds, chia seeds, psyllium husk powder, and salt.

3. Pour in the vegan butter and hot water and mix the ingredients until a dough forms with a gel-like consistency.

4. Line a baking sheet with parchment paper and place the dough on the sheet. Cover the dough with another

parchment paper and with a rolling pin flatten the dough into the baking sheet. Remove the parchment paper on top.

5. Tuck the baking sheet in the oven and bake for 45 minutes, paying close attention to the seeds when the time is almost up. The seeds should have compacted.

6. Turn the oven off and allow the crackers to cool and dry in the oven, about 10 minutes.

7. After, remove the sheet and break the crackers into small pieces. Serve.

NUTRITION VALUES: Calories: 65; Total Fat: 5g; Total Carbs: 3g; Fiber: 1g; Net Carbs: 2g; Protein: 3g

50. MASHED BROCCOLI WITH ROASTED GARLIC

Preparation Time: 5 minutes

Cooking Time: 37 minutes

Servings: 4

INGREDIENTS

- ½ head garlic
- 1 to 2 tbsp of olive oil
- 1 large head broccoli, cut into florets
- Water for boiling, about 3 cups
- 1 tsp salt
- 4 oz. vegan butter
- ¼ tsp dried thyme
- Juice and zest of half a lemon
- 4 tbsp coconut cream
- 4 tbsp olive oil + extra for topping

DIRECTIONS

1. Preheat oven to 400 F.

2. Use a knife to cut a ¼ inch off the top of the garlic cloves, drizzle with the olive oil, and wrap in aluminum foil.

3. Place the wrapped garlic on a baking sheet and roast in the oven for 30 minutes or until the cloves are lightly browned and feel soft when pressed.

4. Remove and set aside when ready.

5. Pour the broccoli into a pot, add the water, and 1 teaspoon of salt. Bring the broccoli to boil over medium heat until tender, about 7 minutes. Then, drain the water and transfer the broccoli to a large bowl.

6. Add the vegan butter, thyme, lemon juice and zest, coconut cream, and olive oil. Use an immersion blender to puree the ingredients until smooth and nice.

7. Spoon the mash into serving bowls and garnish with some olive oil.

8. Serve with grilled eggplants.

NUTRITION VALUES: Calories: 376; Total Fat: 33g; Total Carbs: 8g; Fiber: 2g; Net Carbs: 6g; Protein: 11g

51. KENTUCKY BAKED CAULIFLOWER WITH MASHED PARSNIPS

Preparation Time: 5 minutes

Cooking Time: 30 minutes

Servings: 6

INGREDIENTS

- ½ cup unsweetened almond milk
- ¼ cup coconut flour
- ¼ tsp cayenne pepper
- 1 tsp salt
- ½ cup almond breadcrumbs
- ½ cup shredded vegan cheese
- 30 oz. cauliflower florets
- Mashed Parsnip
- 1 lb medium sized parsnips, peeled and quartered
- 3 tbsp melted vegan butter
- A pinch nutmeg
- 1 tsp cumin powder
- 1 cup coconut cream
- Salt to taste
- Water for boiling
- 2 tbsp sesame oil

DIRECTIONS

For the baked cauliflower

1. Preheat the oven to 425 F and line a baking sheet with parchment paper.

2. In a small bowl, combine the almond milk, coconut flour, and cayenne pepper. In another bowl, mix the salt, breadcrumbs, and vegan cheese. Dip each cauliflower floret into the milk mixture, coating properly, and then into the cheese mixture.

3. Place the breaded cauliflower on the baking sheet and bake in the oven for 30 minutes, turning once after 15 minutes.

For the parsnip mash

1. Make slightly salted water in a saucepan and add the parsnips. Bring to boil over medium heat for 10 to 15 minutes or until the parsnips are fork tender. Drain the parsnips through a colander and transfer to a bowl.

2. Add the melted vegan butter, cumin powder, nutmeg, and coconut cream. Puree the ingredients using an immersion blender until smooth.

3. Spoon the parsnip mash into serving plates and drizzle with some sesame oil. Serve with the baked cauliflower when ready.

NUTRITION VALUES: Calories: 385; Total Fat: 35g; Total Carbs: 12g; Fiber: 4g; Net Carbs: 8g; Protein: 6g

52. BUTTERED CARROT NOODLES WITH KALE

Preparation Time: 5 minutes

Cooking Time: 10 minutes

Servings: 4

INGREDIENTS

- 2 large carrots
- ¼ cup vegetable broth
- 4 tbsp vegan butter
- 1 garlic clove, minced
- 1 cup chopped kale
- ¼ tsp salt
- ¼ tsp freshly ground black pepper

DIRECTIONS

1. Peel the carrots with a slicer and run both through a spiralizer to form noodles.

2. Pour the vegetable broth into a saucepan and add the carrot noodles. Simmer (over low heat) the carrots for 3 minutes. Strain through a colander and set the vegetables aside.

3. Place a large skillet over medium heat and melt the vegan butter. Add the garlic and sauté until softened and put in the kale; cook until wilted.

4. Pour the carrots into the pan, season with the salt and black pepper, and stir-fry for 3 to 4 minutes.

5. Spoon the vegetables into a bowl and serve with pan-grilled tofu.

NUTRITION VALUES: Calories: 335; Total Fat: 28g; Total Carbs: 14g; Fiber: 6g; Net Carbs: 8g; Protein: 6g

53. BAKED SPICY EGGPLANT

Preparation Time: 5 minutes

Cooking Time: 25 minutes

Servings: 4

INGREDIENTS

- 2 large eggplants
- Salt and freshly ground black pepper
- 2 tbsp vegan butter
- 1 tsp red chili flakes
- 4 oz. raw ground almonds

DIRECTIONS

1. Preheat the oven to 400 F.

2. Cut off the head of the eggplants and slice the body into 2-inch rounds. Season with salt and black pepper and arrange on a parchment paper-lined baking sheet.

3. Drop thin slices of the vegan butter on each eggplant slice, sprinkle with red chili flakes, and bake in the oven for 20 minutes.

4. Slide the baking sheet out and sprinkle with the almonds. Roast further for 5 minutes or until golden brown. Dish the eggplants and serve with arugula salad.

NUTRITION VALUES: Calories: 230; Total Fat: 16g; Total Carbs: 8g; Fiber: 4g; Net Carbs: 4g; Protein: 14g

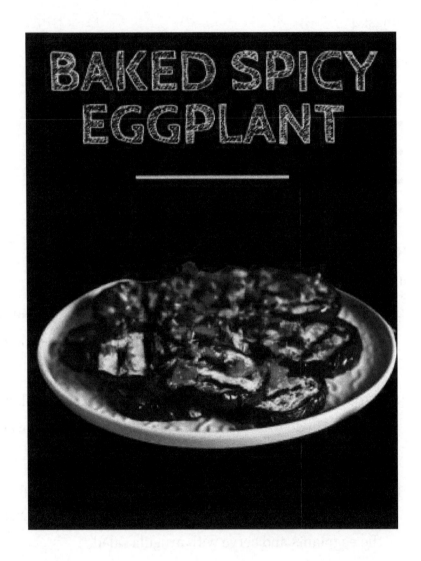

54. SPICY PISTACHIO DIP

Preparation Time: 5 minutes

Servings: 4

INGREDIENTS

- 3 oz. toasted pistachios + a little for garnishing
- 3 tbsp coconut cream
- ¼ cup water
- Juice of half a lemon
- ½ tsp smoked paprika
- Cayenne pepper to taste
- ½ tsp salt
- ½ cup olive oil

DIRECTIONS

1. Pour the pistachios, coconut cream, water, lemon juice, paprika, cayenne pepper, and salt. Puree the ingredients on high speed until smooth.

2. Add the olive oil and puree a little further. Manage the consistency of the dip by adding more oil or water.

3. Spoon the dip into little bowls, garnish with some pistachios, and serve with julienned celery and carrots.

NUTRITION VALUES: Calories: 220; Total Fat: 19g; Total Carbs: 7g; Fiber: 2g; Net Carbs: 5g; Protein: 6g

55. __PARMESAN CROUTONS WITH ROSEMARY TOMATO SOUP__

Preparation Time: 10 minutes

Cooking Time: 1 hour 15 minutes

Servings: 6

INGREDIENTS

Parmesan Croutons:

- 3 tbsp flax seed powder + 9 tbsp water
- 1¼ cups almond flour
- 2 tsp baking powder
- 5 tbsp psyllium husk powder
- 1 tsp salt
- 1¼ cups boiling water
- 2 tsp plain vinegar
- Olive oil for greasing

Parmesan topping

- 3 oz. vegan butter
- 2 oz. grated vegan parmesan cheese
- Rosemary Tomato Soup
- 2 lb fresh ripe tomatoes
- 4 cloves garlic, peeled only
- 1 small white onion, diced
- 1 small red bell pepper, seeded and diced
- 3 tbsp olive oil

- 1 cup coconut cream
- ½ tsp dried rosemary
- ½ tsp dried oregano
- 2 tbsp chopped fresh basil
- Salt and freshly ground black pepper to taste
- Basil leaves to garnish

DIRECTIONS

For the parmesan croutons:

1. In a medium bowl, mix the flax seed powder with 2/3 cup of water and set aside to soak for 5 minutes. Preheat the oven to 350 F and line a baking sheet with parchment paper.

2. In another bowl, combine the almond flour, baking powder, psyllium husk powder, and salt.

3. When the flax egg is ready, mix in the boiling water and plain vinegar. Then, add the flour mixture and whisk for 30 seconds just to be well combined but not overly mixed.

4. Grease your hands with some olive oil and form 8 flat pieces out of the dough. Place the flattened dough on the baking sheet while leaving enough room between each to allow rising. Bake the dough for 40 minutes or until crispy.

5. Remove the croutons to cool and break them into halves.

6. Mix the vegan butter with vegan parmesan cheese and spread the mixture in the inner parts of the croutons.

7. Increase the oven's temperature to 450 F and bake the croutons further for 5 minutes or until golden brown and crispier.

For the tomato soup:
1. In a baking pan, add the tomatoes, garlic, onion, red bell pepper, and drizzle with the olive oil.

2. Roast the vegetables in the oven for 25 minutes and after broil for 3 to 4 minutes until some of the tomatoes are slightly charred.

3. Transfer the vegetables to a blender and add the coconut cream, rosemary, oregano, basil, salt, and black pepper. Puree the ingredients on high speed until smooth and creamy. If the soup is too thick, add a little water to lighten the texture.

4. 1Pour the soup into serving bowls, drop some croutons on top, garnish with some basil leaves, and serve.

NUTRITION VALUES: Calories: 434; Total Fat: 38g; Total Carbs: 12g; Fiber: 6g; Net Carbs: 6g; Protein: 11g

56. **PARIKA ROASTED NUTS**

Preparation Time: 3 minutes

Cooking Time: 7 minutes

Servings: 4

INGREDIENTS

- 8 oz. walnuts and pecans
- 1 tsp salt
- 1 tbsp coconut oil
- 1 tsp cumin powder
- 1 tsp paprika powder

DIRECTIONS

1. In a bowl, mix the walnuts, pecans, salt, coconut oil, cumin powder, and paprika powder until the nuts are well coated with spice and oil.

2. Pour the mixture into a frying pan and toast over medium heat while stirring continually.

3. Once the nuts are fragrant and brown, transfer to a bowl. Allow to cool and serve with a chilled berry juice.

NUTRITION VALUES: Calories: 290; Total Fat: 27g; Total Carbs: 6g; Fiber: 3g; Net Carbs: 3g; Protein: 6g

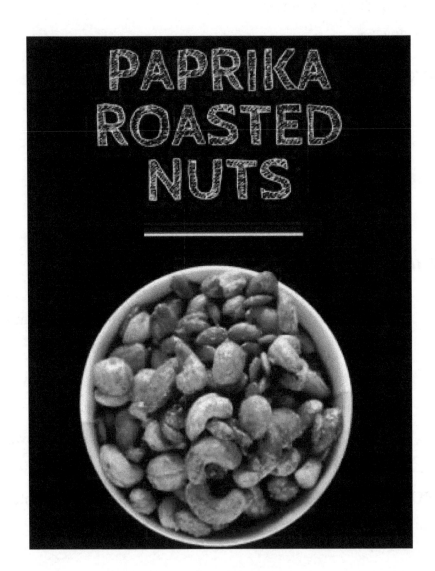

57. SPINACH CHIPS WITH GUACAMOLE HUMMUS

Preparation Time: 12 minutes

Cooking Time: 15 minutes

Servings: 4

INGREDIENTS

Spinach Chips:

- ½ cup baby spinach
- 1 tbsp olive oil
- ½ tsp plain vinegar
- Salt to taste

Guacamole Hummus:

- 3 large avocados, ripe and soft
- ½ cup freshly chopped parsley + extra for garnishing
- ½ cup vegan butter
- ¼ cup pumpkin seeds
- ¼ cup sesame paste
- Juice from ½ lemon
- 1 garlic clove, minced
- ½ tsp coriander powder
- Salt and black pepper to taste

DIRECTIONS

Spinach Chips:

1. Preheat the oven to 300 F.

2. Rinse the spinach under running water and pat dry with a paper towel(s). Put the spinach in a bowl and toss with olive oil, plain vinegar, and salt.

3. After, arrange the spinach on a parchment paper-lined baking sheet and bake in the oven until the leaves are crispy but not burned, about 15 minutes. Toss a few times to ensure an even bake.

Guacamole Hummus:

1. Use a knife to cut the avocado in half lengthwise, take out the pit, and scoop the flesh into the bowl of a food processor.

2. Add the parsley, vegan butter, pumpkin seeds, sesame paste, lemon juice, garlic, coriander powder, salt, and black pepper. Puree the ingredients until smooth. If too thick, mix in some more olive oil or water. Spoon the hummus into a bowl and garnish with some parsley.

3. Serve the guacamole hummus with the spinach chips.

NUTRITION VALUES: Calories: 473; Total Fat: 45g; Total Carbs: 8g; Fiber: 5g; Net Carbs: 3g; Protein: 8g

VEGETABLES

58. GARLIC TOMATOES

Preparation Time: 60 minutes

Servings: 4

INGREDIENTS

- 4 garlic cloves; crushed
- 1 lb. mixed cherry tomatoes
- 3 thyme springs; chopped
- A pinch of sea salt
- Black pepper to the taste
- 1/4 Cup Olive Oil

DIRECTIONS

1. In a baking dish, mix tomatoes with a pinch of sea salt, black pepper, olive oil and thyme, toss to coat, place in the oven at 325 °F and bake for 50 minutes. Divide tomatoes and pan juices between plates and serve.

NUTRITION VALUES: Calories: 100; Fat: 0g; Fiber: 1g; Carbs: 1g; Protein: 6g

Garlic
Tomatoes

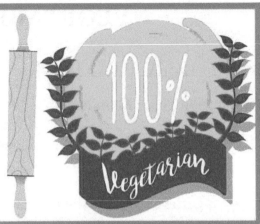

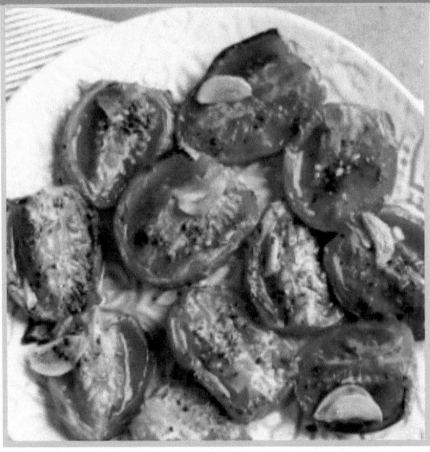

59. GRILLED ARTICHOKES

Preparation Time: 35 minutes

Servings: 4

INGREDIENTS

- 2 artichokes; trimmed and halved
- Juice of 1 lemon
- 1 tbsp. lemon zest grated
- 1 rosemary spring; chopped
- 2 tbsp. olive oil
- A pinch of sea salt
- Black Pepper To The Taste

DIRECTIONS

1. Put water in a pot, add a pinch of salt and lemon juice, bring to a boil over medium high heat, add artichokes, boil for 15 minutes, drain and leave them to cool down.
2. Drizzle olive oil over them, season with black pepper to the taste, sprinkle lemon zest and rosemary, stir well and place them on your preheated grill.
3. Grill artichokes over medium high heat for 5 minutes on each side, divide them between plates and serve.

NUTRITION VALUES: Calories: 120; Fat: 1g; Fiber: 2g; Carbs: 6g; Protein: 7g

Grilled
Artichokes

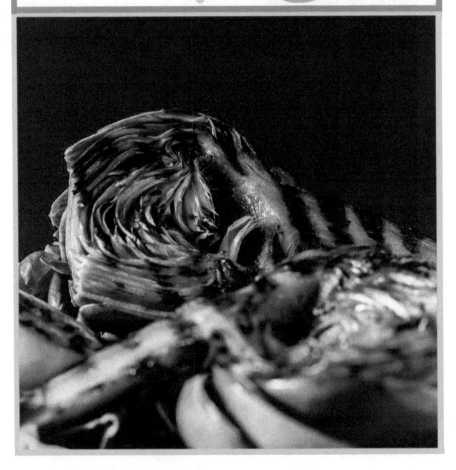

60. PORK STUFFED BELL PEPPERS

Preparation Time: 36 minutes

Servings: 4

INGREDIENTS

- 1 tsp. Cajun spice
- 1 lb. pork; ground
- 1 tbsp. olive oil
- 1 tbsp. tomato paste
- 6 garlic cloves; minced
- 1 yellow onion; chopped
- 4 big bell peppers; tops cut off and seeds removed
- A pinch of sea salt
- Black Pepper To The Taste

DIRECTIONS

1. Heat up a pan with the oil over medium high heat, add garlic and onion, stir and cook for 4 minutes.
2. Add meat, stir and cook for 10 minutes more.
3. Add a pinch of salt, black pepper, tomato paste and Cajun seasoning, stir and cook for 3 minutes more.
4. Stuff bell peppers with this mix, place them on preheated grill over medium high heat, grill for 3 minutes on each side, divide between plates and serve.

NUTRITION VALUES: Calories: 140; Fat: 3g; Fiber: 2g; Carbs: 3g; Protein: 10g

61. CARROTS AND LIME

Preparation Time: 40 minutes

Servings: 6

INGREDIENTS

- 1¼ lbs. baby carrots
- 3 tbsp. ghee; melted
- 8 garlic cloves; minced
- A pinch of sea salt
- Black pepper to the taste
- Zest of 2 limes; grated
- 1/2 Tsp. Chili Powder

DIRECTIONS

1. In a bowl; mix baby carrots with ghee, garlic, a pinch of salt, black pepper to the taste and chili powder and stir well.
2. Spread carrots on a lined baking sheet, place in the oven at 400 °F and roast for 15 minutes.
3. Take carrots out of the oven, shake baking sheet, place in the oven again and roast for 15 minutes more. Divide between plates and serve with lime on top.

NUTRITION VALUES: Calories: 100; Fat: 1g; Fiber: 1g; Carbs: 1g; Protein: 7g

Carrots And Lime

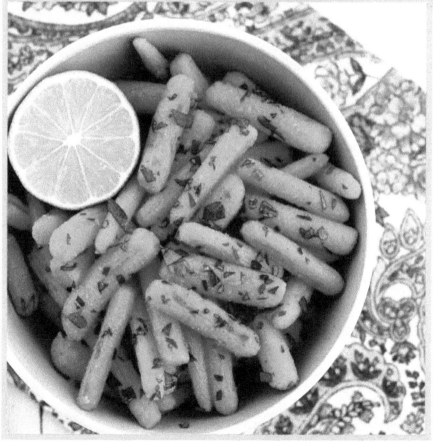

62.   EGGPLANT CASSEROLE

Preparation Time: 60 minutes

Servings: 4

INGREDIENTS

- 2 eggplants; sliced
- 3 tbsp. olive oil
- 1 lb. beef; ground
- 1 garlic clove; minced
- 3/4 cup tomato sauce
- 1/2 bunch basil; chopped
- A pinch of sea salt
- Black Pepper To The Taste

DIRECTIONS

1. Heat up a pan with 1 tbsp. oil over medium high heat, add eggplant slices, cook for 5 minutes on each side, transfer them to paper towels, drain grease and leave them aside.
2. Heat up another pan with the rest of the oil over medium high heat, add garlic, stir and cook for 1 minute.
3. Add beef, stir and cook for 5 minutes more.
4. Add tomato sauce, stir and cook for 5 minutes more.
5. Add a pinch of sea salt and black pepper, stir; take off heat and mix with basil.

6. Place one layer of eggplant slices into a baking dish, add one layer of beef mix and repeat with the rest of the eggplant slices and beef.

7. Place in the oven at 350 °F and bake for 30 minutes. Leave eggplant casserole to cool down, slice and serve.

NUTRITION VALUES: Calories: 342; Fat: 23g; Fiber: 7g; Carbs: 10g; Protein: 23g

63. __WARM WATERCRESS MIX__

Preparation Time: 20 minutes

Servings: 4

INGREDIENTS

- 1 lb. watercress; chopped
- 1/4 cup olive oil
- 1 garlic clove; cut in halves
- 1 bacon slice; cooked and crumbled
- 1/4 cup hazelnuts; chopped
- Black pepper to the taste
- 1/4 Cup Pine Nuts

DIRECTIONS

1. Heat up a pan with the oil over medium heat, add garlic clove halves, cook for 2 minutes and discard.
2. Heat up the pan with the garlic oil again over medium heat, add hazelnuts and pine nuts, stir and cook for 6 minutes.
3. Add bacon, black pepper to the taste and watercress, stir; cook for 2 minutes, divide between plates and serve right away.

NUTRITION VALUES: Calories: 100; Fat: 1g; Fiber: 2g; Carbs: 2g; Protein: 6g

Warm
Watercress
Mix

100%
Vegetarian

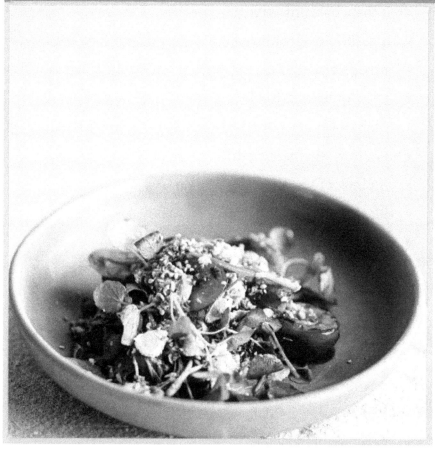

64. ARTICHOKES DISH

Preparation Time: 60 minutes

Servings: 4

INGREDIENTS

- 16 mushrooms; sliced
- 1/3 cup tamari sauce
- 1/3 cup olive oil
- 4 tbsp. balsamic vinegar
- 4 garlic cloves; minced
- 1 tbsp. lemon juice
- 1 tsp. oregano; dried
- 1 tsp. rosemary; dried
- 1/2 tbsp. thyme; dried
- A pinch of sea salt
- Black pepper to the taste
- 1 sweet onion; chopped
- 1 jar artichoke hearts
- 4 cups spinach
- 1 tbsp. coconut oil
- 1 tsp. garlic; minced
- 1 cauliflower head; florets separated
- 1/2 cup veggie stock
- 1 tsp. garlic powder
- A Pinch Of Nutmeg; Ground

DIRECTIONS

- In a bowl; mix vinegar with tamari sauce, lemon juice, 4 garlic cloves, olive oil, oregano, rosemary, thyme, a pinch of salt, black pepper and mushrooms, toss to coat well and leave aside for 30 minutes.
- Transfer these to a lined baking sheet and bake them in the oven at 350 °F for 30 minutes.
- In your food processor, mix cauliflower with a pinch of sea salt and black pepper and pulse until you obtain your rice.
- Heat up a pan over medium high heat, add cauliflower rice, toast for 2 minutes, add nutmeg, garlic powder, black pepper and stock, stir and cook until stock evaporated.
- Heat up a pan with the coconut oil over medium heat, add onion, artichokes, 1 tsp. garlic and spinach, stir and cook for a few minutes. Divide cauliflower rice on plates, top with artichokes and mushrooms and serve.

NUTRITION VALUES: Calories: 200; Fat: 3g; Fiber: 2g; Carbs: 7g; Protein: 18g

65. CUCUMBER NOODLES AND SHRIMP

Preparation Time: 25 minutes

Servings: 4

INGREDIENTS

- 1 tbsp. Paleo tamari sauce
- 3 tbsp. coconut aminos
- 1 tbsp. sriracha
- 1 tbsp. balsamic vinegar
- 1/2 cup warm water
- 1 tbsp. honey
- 3 tbsp. lemongrass; chopped
- 1 tbsp. ginger; dried
- 1 lb. shrimp; peeled and deveined
- 1 Tbsp. Olive Oil

For the cucumber noodles:

- 2 cucumbers; cut with a spiralizer
- 1 carrot; cut into thin matchsticks
- 1/4 cup balsamic vinegar
- 1/4 cup ghee; melted
- 1/4 cup peanuts; roasted
- 2 tbsp. sriracha sauce
- 1 tbsp. coconut aminos
- 1 tbsp. ginger; grated
- A Handful Mint; Chopped

DIRECTIONS

1. In a bowl; mix 3 tbsp. coconut aminos with 1 tbsp. vinegar, 1 tbsp. tamari, 1 tbsp. sriracha, warm water, honey, lemongrass, 1 tbsp. ginger, 1 tbsp. olive oil and whisk well.
2. Add shrimp, toss to coat and leave aside for 20 minutes.
3. Heat up your grill over medium high heat, add shrimp, cook them for 3 minutes on each side and transfer to a bowl.
4. In a bowl; mix cucumber noodles with carrot, ghee, 1/4 cup vinegar, 2 tbsp. Sriracha, 1 tbsp. coconut aminos, 1 tbsp. ginger, peanuts and mint and stir well. Divide cucumber noodles on plates, top with shrimp and serve.

NUTRITION VALUES: Calories: 140; Fat: 1g; Fiber: 2g; Carbs: 3g; Protein: 8g

66. BAKED EGGPLANT

Preparation Time: 40 minutes

Servings: 3

INGREDIENTS

- 2 eggplants; sliced
- A pinch of sea salt
- Black pepper to the taste
- 1 cup almonds; ground
- 1 tsp. garlic; minced
- 2 Tsp. Olive Oil

DIRECTIONS

1. Grease a baking dish with some of the oil and arrange eggplant slices on it.
2. Season them with a pinch of salt and some black pepper and leave them aside for 10 minutes.
3. In your food processor, mix almonds with the rest of the oil, garlic, a pinch of salt and black pepper and blend well.
4. Spread this over eggplant slices, place in the oven at 425 °F and bake for 30 minutes. Divide between plates and serve.

NUTRITION VALUES: Calories: 140; Fat: 1g; Fiber: 1g; Carbs: 3g; Protein: 15g

67. PURPLE CARROTS

Preparation Time: 1 hour 10 minutes

Servings: 2

INGREDIENTS

- 6 purple carrots; peeled
- A drizzle of olive oil
- 2 tbsp. sesame seeds paste
- 6 tbsp. water
- 3 tbsp. lemon juice
- 1 garlic clove; minced
- A pinch of sea salt
- Black pepper to the taste
- White And Sesame Seeds

DIRECTIONS

1. Arrange purple carrots on a lined baking sheet, sprinkle a pinch of salt, black pepper and a drizzle of oil, place in the oven at 350 °F and bake for 1 hour.
2. Meanwhile; in your food processor, mix sesame seeds paste with water, lemon juice, garlic, a pinch of sea salt and black pepper and pulse really well.
3. Spread this over carrots, toss gently, divide between plates and sprinkle sesame seeds on top.

NUTRITION VALUES: Calories: 100; Fat: 1g; Fiber: 1g; Carbs: 5g; Protein: 10g

Purple Carrots

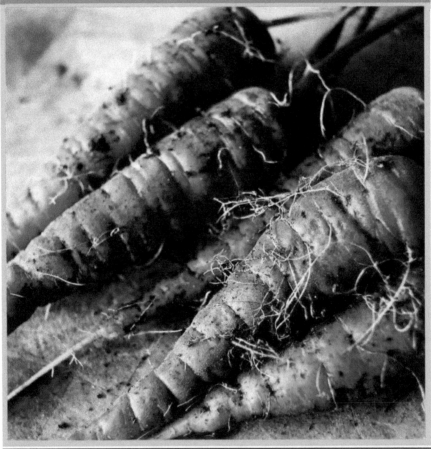

68.   STUFFED WITH BEEF

Preparation Time: 1 hour 5 minutes

Servings: 2

INGREDIENTS

- 1 lb. beef; ground
- 1 tsp. coriander; ground
- 1 onion; chopped
- 3 garlic cloves; minced
- 2 tbsp. coconut oil
- 1 tbsp. ginger; grated
- 1/2 tsp. cumin
- 1/2 tsp. turmeric
- 1 tbsp. hot curry powder
- A pinch of sea salt
- 1 egg
- 4 bell peppers; cut in halves and seeds removed
- 1/3 cup raisins
- 1/3 Cup Walnuts; Chopped

DIRECTIONS

1. Heat up a pan with the oil over medium high heat, add onion, stir and cook for 4 minutes.
2. Add garlic, stir and cook for 1 minute.
3. Add beef, stir and cook for 10 minutes.

4. Add coriander, ginger, cumin, curry powder, a pinch of salt and turmeric and stir well.

5. Add walnuts and raisins, stir take off heat and mix with egg.

6. Divide this mix into pepper halves, place them on a lined baking sheet, place in the oven at 350 °F and bake for 40 minutes. Divide between plates and serve.

NUTRITION VALUES: Calories: 240; Fat: 4g; Fiber: 3g; Carbs: 7g; Protein: 12g

69. __CARROT HASH__

Preparation Time: 55 minutes

Servings: 4

INGREDIENTS

- 1 tbsp. olive oil
- 6 bacon slices; chopped
- 3 cups carrots; chopped
- 3/4 lb. beef; ground
- 1 yellow onion; chopped
- A pinch of sea salt
- Black pepper to the taste
- 2 Scallions; Chopped

DIRECTIONS

1. Place carrots on a lined baking sheet, drizzle the oil, season with a pinch of salt and some black pepper, toss to coat, place in the oven at 425 °F and bake for 25 minutes.
2. Meanwhile; heat up a pan over medium high heat, add bacon and fry for a couple of minutes.
3. Add onion and beef and some black pepper, stir and cook for 7-8 minutes more.
4. Take carrots out of the oven, add them to the beef and bacon mix, stir and cook for 10 minutes. Sprinkle scallions on top, divide between plates and serve.

NUTRITION VALUES: Calories: 160; Fat: 2g; Fiber: 1g; Carbs: 2g; Protein: 12g

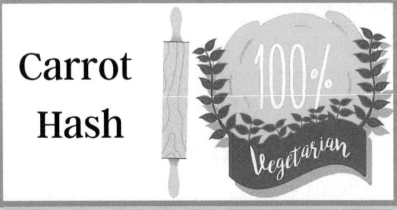

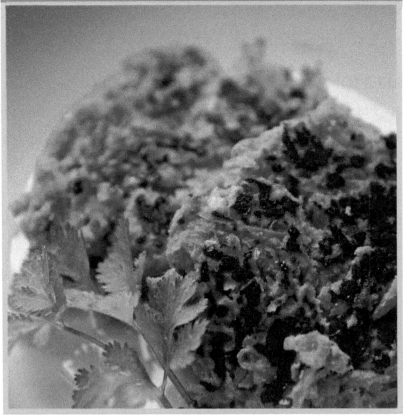

70. STUFFED POBLANOS

Preparation Time: 50 minutes

Servings: 4

INGREDIENTS

- 2 tsp. garlic; minced
- 1 white onion; chopped
- 10 poblano peppers; one side of them sliced and reserved
- 1 tbsp. olive oil
- Cooking spray
- 8 oz. mushrooms; chopped
- A pinch of sea salt
- Black pepper to the taste
- 1/2 Cup Cilantro; Chopped

DIRECTIONS

1. Place poblano boats in a baking dish which you've sprayed with some cooking spray.
2. Heat up a pan with the oil over medium high heat, add chopped poblano pieces, onion and mushrooms, stir and cook for 5 minutes.
3. Add garlic, cilantro, salt and black pepper, stir and cook for 2 minutes.
4. Divide this into poblano boats, introduce them in the oven at 375 °F and bake for 30 minutes. Divide between plates and serve.

NUTRITION VALUES: Calories: 150; Fat: 3g; Fiber: 2g; Carbs: 4g; Protein: 10g

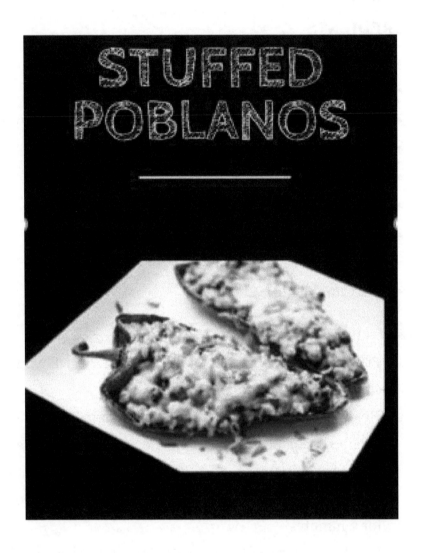

71. TOMATO QUICHE

Preparation Time: 30 minutes

Servings: 2

INGREDIENTS

- 1 bunch basil; chopped
- 4 eggs
- 1 garlic clove; minced
- A pinch of sea salt
- Black pepper to the taste
- 1/2 cup cherry tomatoes; halved
- 1/4 Cup Almond Cheese

DIRECTIONS

1. In a bowl; mix eggs with a pinch of sea salt, black pepper, almond cheese and basil and whisk well.
2. Pour this into a baking dish, arrange tomatoes on top, place in the oven at 350 °F and bake for 20 minutes. Leave quiche to cool down, slice and serve.

NUTRITION VALUES: Calories: 140; Fat: 1g; Fiber: 1g; Carbs: 2g; Protein: 10g

72. **LIVER STUFFED PEPPERS**

Preparation Time: 25 minutes

Servings: 4

INGREDIENTS

- 4 bacon slices; chopped
- 1 white onion; chopped
- 1/2 lb. chicken livers; chopped
- 4 garlic cloves; chopped
- 4 bell peppers; tops cut off and seeds removed
- A pinch of sea salt
- Black pepper to the taste
- 1/2 tsp. lemon zest; grated
- 1/4 tsp. thyme; chopped
- 1/4 tsp. dill; chopped
- A drizzle of olive oil
- A Handful Parsley; Chopped

DIRECTIONS

1. Heat up a pan over medium heat, add bacon, stir and cook for 2 minutes.
2. Add onion and garlic, stir and cook for 2 minutes.
3. Add livers, a pinch of salt and black pepper, stir; cook for 5 minutes and take off heat.
4. Transfer this to your food processor, blend very well, transfer to a bowl and aside for 10 minutes.

5. Add thyme, oil, parsley, lemon zest and dill, stir well and Stuff each bell pepper with this mix. Serve right away.

NUTRITION VALUES: Calories: 150; Fat: 3g; Fiber: 2g; Carbs: 5g; Protein: 12g

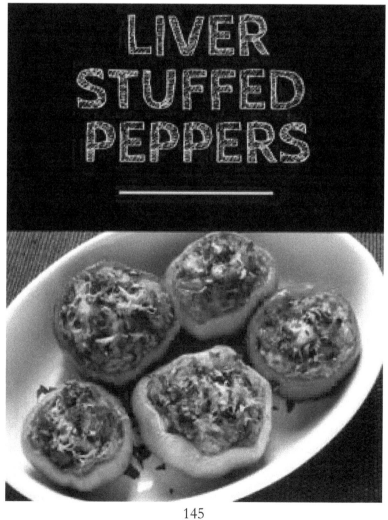

73. **STUFFED PORTOBELLO MUSHROOMS**

Preparation Time: 30 minutes

Servings: 4

INGREDIENTS

- 10 basil leaves
- 1 cup baby spinach
- 3 garlic cloves; chopped
- 1 cup almonds; roughly chopped
- 1 tbsp. parsley
- 2 tbsp. Nutritional yeast
- 1/4 cup olive oil
- 8 cherry tomatoes; halved
- A pinch of sea salt
- Black pepper to the taste
- 4 Portobello Mushrooms; Stem Removed and Chopped

DIRECTIONS

1. In your food processor, mix basil with spinach, garlic, almonds, parsley, Nutritional yeast, oil, a pinch of salt, black pepper to the taste and mushroom stems and blend well.

2. Stuff each mushroom with this mix, place them on a lined baking sheet, place in the oven at 400 °F and bake for 20 minutes. Divide between plates and serve right away.

NUTRITION VALUES: Calories: 145; Fat: 3g; Fiber: 2g; Carbs: 6g; Protein: 17g

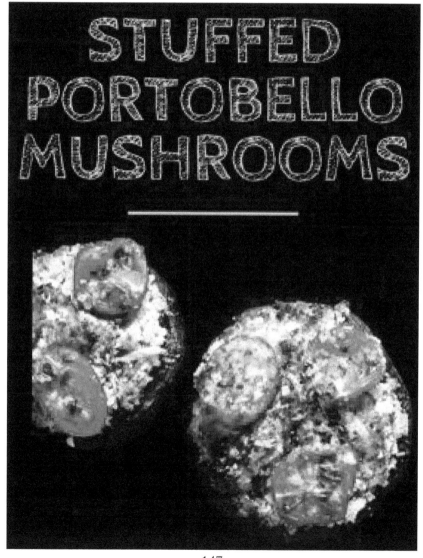

74. <u>ZUCCHINI NOODLES AND PESTO</u>

Preparation Time: 20 minutes

Servings: 4

INGREDIENTS

- 6 zucchinis; trimmed and cut with a spiralizer
- 1 cup basil
- 1 avocado; pitted and peeled
- A pinch of sea salt
- Black pepper to the taste
- 3 garlic cloves; chopped
- 1/4 cup olive oil
- 2 tbsp. olive oil
- 1 lb. shrimp; peeled and deveined
- 1/4 cup pistachios
- 2 tbsp. lemon juice
- 2 Tsp. Old Bay Seasoning

DIRECTIONS

1. In a bowl; mix zucchini noodles with a pinch of sea salt and some black pepper, leave aside for 10 minutes and squeeze well.
2. In your food processor, mix pistachios with black pepper, basil, avocado, lemon juice and a pinch of salt and blend well.
3. Add 1/4 cup oil, blend again and leave aside for now.

4. Heat up a pan with 1 tbsp. oil over medium high heat, add garlic, stir and cook for 1 minute.

5. Add shrimp and old bay seasoning, stir; cook for 4 minutes and transfer to a bowl.

6. Heat up the same pan with the rest of the oil over medium high heat, add zucchini noodles, stir and cook for 3 minutes.

7. Divide on plates, add pesto on top and toss to coat well. top with shrimp and serve.

NUTRITION VALUES: Calories: 140; Fat: 1g; Fiber: 1g; Carbs: 5g; Protein: 14g

75. SPAGHETTI SQUASH AND TOMATOES

Preparation Time: 60 minutes

Servings: 4

INGREDIENTS

- 1/4 cup pine nuts
- 2 cups basil; chopped
- 1 spaghetti squash; halved lengthwise and seedless
- Black pepper to the taste
- A pinch of sea salt
- 1 tsp. garlic; minced
- 1½ tbsp. olive oil
- 1 cup mixed cherry tomatoes; halved
- 1/2 cup olive oil
- 2 Garlic Cloves; Minced

DIRECTIONS

1. Place spaghetti squash halves on a lined baking sheet, place in the oven at 375 °F and bake for 40 minutes.
2. Leave squash to cool down and make your spaghetti out of the flesh.
3. In your food processor, mix pine nuts with a pinch of salt, basil and 2 garlic cloves and blend well.
4. Add 1/2 cup olive oil, blend again well and transfer to a bowl.

5. Heat up a pan with 1½ tbsp. oil over medium high heat, add tomatoes, a pinch of salt, some black pepper and 1 tsp. garlic, stir and cook for 2 minutes. Divide spaghetti squash on plates, add tomatoes and the basil pesto on top.

NUTRITION VALUES: Calories: 150; Fat: 1g; Fiber: 2g; Carbs: 4g; Protein: 12g

76. **DAIKON ROLLS**

Preparation Time: 15 minutes

Servings: 4

INGREDIENTS

- 1/2 cup pumpkin seeds
- 2 green onions; chopped
- 1/2 bunch cilantro; roughly chopped
- 2 tbsp. avocado oil
- 1 tbsp. lime juice
- 2 tsp. water
- A pinch of sea salt
- Black pepper to the taste
- 2 daikon radishes; sliced lengthwise into long strips
- 1 small cucumber; cut into matchsticks
- 1/2 avocado; pitted, peeled and sliced
- Handful Microgreens

DIRECTIONS

1. In your food processor, mix pumpkin seeds with a pinch of sea salt, pepper, cilantro and green onions and blend very well.

2. Add avocado oil gradually and lime juice and blend very well again. Add water and blend some more.

3. Spread this on each daikon slice, add cucumber matchsticks, avocado slices and micro greens, roll them, seal edges, divide between plates and serve.

NUTRITION VALUES: Calories: 140; Fat: 0g; Carbs: 23g; Fiber: 0g; Protein: 0

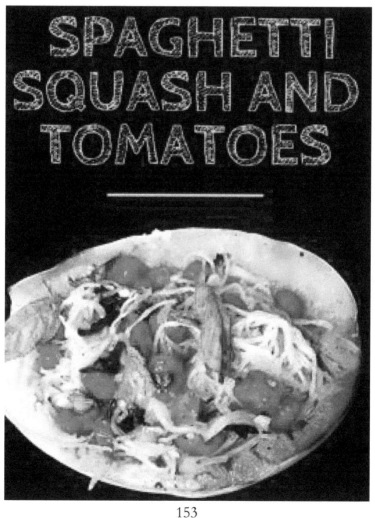

77. <u>GLAZED CARROTS</u>

Preparation Time: 25 minutes

Servings: 4

INGREDIENTS

- 1 lb. carrots; sliced
- 1 tbsp. coconut oil
- 1 tbsp. ghee
- 1/2 cup pineapple juice
- 1 tsp. ginger; grated
- 1/2 tbsp. maple syrup
- 1/2 tsp. nutmeg
- 1 Tbsp. Parsley; Chopped

DIRECTIONS

1. Heat up a pan with the ghee and the oil over medium high heat, add ginger, stir and cook for 2 minutes.
2. Add carrots, stir and cook for 5 minutes.
3. Add pineapple juice, maple syrup and nutmeg, stir and cook for 5 minutes more. Add parsley, stir; cook for 3 minutes, divide between plates and serve.

NUTRITION VALUES: Calories: 100; Fat: 0.5g; Fiber: 1g; Carbs: 3g; Protein: 7g

GLAZED CARROTS

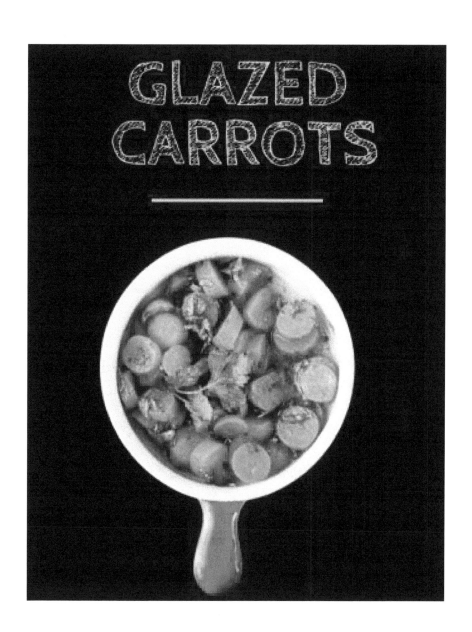

78. CAULIFLOWER PIZZA

Preparation Time: 40 minutes

Servings: 6

INGREDIENTS

- 1½ cups mashed cauliflower
- A pinch of sea salt
- Black pepper to the taste
- 1/2 cup almond meal
- 1½ tbsp. flax seed; ground
- 2/3 cup water
- 1/2 tsp. oregano; dried
- 1/2 tsp. garlic powder
- Pizza sauce for serving
- Spinach leaves; chopped and already cooked for serving
- Mushrooms; Sliced And Cooked For Serving

DIRECTIONS

1. In a bowl; mix flax seed with water and stir well.
2. In a bowl; mix cauliflower with almond meal, flax seed mix, a pinch of sea salt, pepper, oregano and garlic powder, stir well, shape small pizza crusts, spread them on a lined baking sheet and bake them in the oven at 420 °F and bake for 15 minutes.
3. Take pizzas out of the oven, spread pizza sauce, spinach and mushrooms on them, introduce in the oven again

and bake 10 more minutes. Divide between plates and serve.

NUTRITION VALUES: Calories: 150; Fat: 8g; Carbs: 20g; Fiber: 1g; Protein: 9g

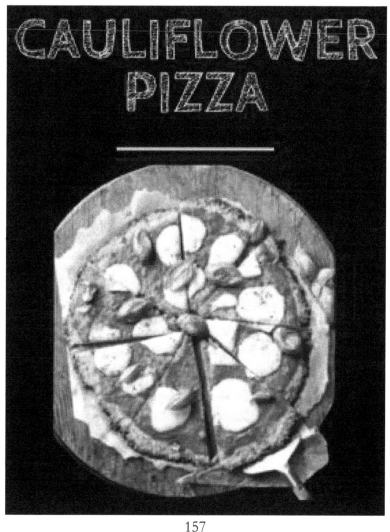

79. **CUCUMBER WRAPS**

Preparation Time: 40 minutes

Servings: 4

INGREDIENTS

For the mayo:

- 1 tbsp. coconut aminos
- 3 tbsp. lemon juice
- 1 cup macadamia nuts
- 1 tbsp. agave
- 1 tsp. caraway seeds
- 1/3 cup dill; chopped
- A pinch of sea salt
- Some Water

For the filling:

- 1 cup alfalfa sprouts
- 1 red bell pepper; cut into thin strips
- 2 carrots; cut into thin matchsticks
- 1 cucumber; cut into thin matchsticks
- 1 cup pea shoots
- 4 Paleo Coconut Wrappers

DIRECTIONS

1. Put macadamia nuts in a bowl; add water to cover, leave aside for 30 minutes and drain well.

2. In your food processor, mix nuts with coconut aminos, lemon juice, agave, caraway seeds, a pinch of salt and dill and blend very well.
3. Add some water and blend again until you obtain a smooth mayo.
4. Divide alfalfa sprouts, bell pepper, carrot, cucumber and pea shoots on each coconut wrappers, spread dill mayo over them, wrap, cut each in half and serve.

NUTRITION VALUES: Calories: 140; Fat: 3g; Fiber: 3g; Carbs: 5g; Protein: 12g

5. Meanwhile; heat up a pan over medium high heat, add bacon and fry for a couple of minutes.
6. Add onion and beef and some black pepper, stir and cook for 7-8 minutes more.
7. Take carrots out of the oven, add them to the beef and bacon mix, stir and cook for 10 minutes. Sprinkle scallions on top, divide between plates and serve.

NUTRITION VALUES: Calories: 160; Fat: 2g; Fiber: 1g; Carbs: 2g; Protein: 12g

SALADS

80. THAI PAPAYA SALAD

Preparation Time: 10 minutes

Servings: 4

NUTRITIONAL VALUES: Calories: 71 Fat: 3 g. Protein: 3 g. Carbs: 9 g.

INGREDIENTS

- 300 grams Green Papaya, shredded
- 100 grams Tomatoes, diced
- 30 grams Roasted Peanuts, chopped
- Chopped Cilantro

For the Dressing:

- ¼ cup Lime Juice
- 2 tbsp Vegan Fish Sauce
- 1 tbsp Erythritol
- 1 clove Garlic, minced
- 1 Red Chili, minced

DIRECTIONS

1. Whisk all ingredients for the dressing in a bowl.
2. Toss in shredded papaya and tomatoes.

3. Top with chopped peanuts and cilantro.

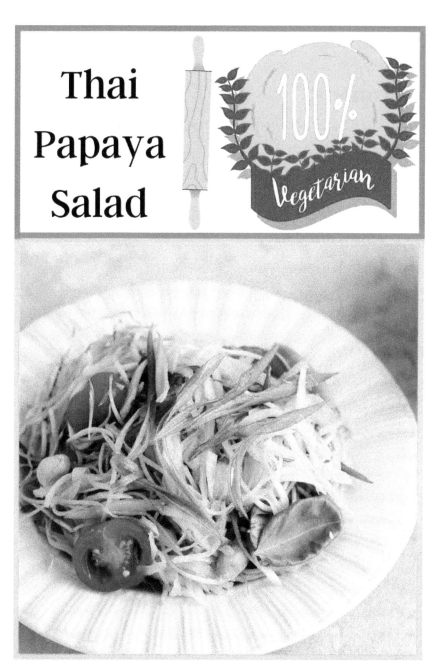

Thai Papaya Salad

100%
Vegetarian

81. STRAWBERRY AND PECAN SALAD

Preparation Time: 10 minutes

Servings: 4

NUTRITIONAL VALUES: Calories: 178 Fat: 16 g. Protein: 2 g Carbs: 9 g.

INGREDIENTS

- 250 grams Strawberries, rough-chopped
- 75 grams Shallots, thinly-sliced
- 30 grams Roasted Pecans, rough-chopped

For the Dressing:

- 3 tbsp Olive Oil
- 1 tbsp Balsamic Vinegar
- ½ tsp Freshly Ground Black Pepper
- ¼ tsp Salt

DIRECTIONS

1. Whisk all ingredients for the dressing in a bowl.
2. Toss in the strawberries, shallots, and pecans.

82. WATERCRESS SLAW IN LIME VINAIGRETTE

Preparation Time: 5 minutes

Servings: 2

NUTRITIONAL VALUES: Calories: 195 Fat: 20 g. Protein: 2 g. Carbs: 3 g.

INGREDIENTS

- 200 grams Watercress

For the Vinaigrette:

- 3 tbsp Olive Oil
- 1 tbsp Lime Juice
- 1 tbsp Minced Shallots
- ¼ tsp Black Pepper
- ¼ tsp Salt

DIRECTIONS

1. Whisk all ingredients for the dressing in a bowl.
2. Toss in the watercress until evenly coated.

83. SPICED BEAN SPROUT SALAD

Preparation Time: 10 minutes

Servings: 4

NUTRITIONAL VALUES: Calories: 142 Fat: 12 g. Protein: 4 g. Carbs: 6 g.

INGREDIENTS

- 300 grams Bean Sprouts
- 70 grams Carrots, thinly sliced
- 70 grams Jicama, thinly sliced
- 1 tbsp Sesame Seeds
- 2 tbsp Chopped Spring Onions

For the Dressing:

- 2 tbsp Rice Wine Vinegar
- 1 tbsp Tamari
- 2 tsp Gochujang
- 1 tbsp Sesame Oil
- 2 tsp Erythritol
- 2 tbsp Olive Oil

DIRECTIONS

1. Whisk all ingredients for the dressing in a bowl.
2. Toss in the bean sprouts, carrots, and jicamas.
3. Top with sesame seeds and spring onions.

Spiced Bean Sprout Salad

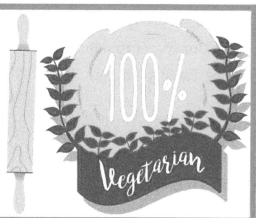

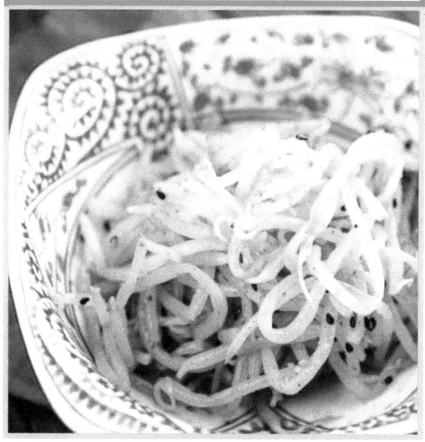

84. GRILLED ASPARAGUS AND MUSHROOM SALAD

Preparation Time: 10 minutes

Cooking Time: 5 minutes

Servings: 4

NUTRITIONAL VALUES: Calories: 159 Fat: 14 g. Protein: 3 g. Carbs: 7 g.

INGREDIENTS

- 200 grams Asparagus
- 200 grams Portobello Mushrooms
- 100 grams Red Onion, cut in half

For the Dressing:

- 1/4 cup Olive Oil
- tbsp Balsamic Vinegar
- 1 tbsp Chopped Fresh Parsley
- pinch of Salt and Pepper to taste

DIRECTIONS

1. Whisk all ingredients for the dressing in a bowl.
2. Transfer half of the dressing in a separate bowl and set aside.
3. Toss asparagus, mushrooms, and red onion in half of the dressing.
4. Cook the vegetables on a hot grill.
5. Roughly chop the grilled veggies and toss in the reserved dressing.

85. VEGAN COLESLAW

Preparation Time: 1 hour

Cooking Time:

Servings: 8

NUTRITIONAL VALUES: Calories: 271 Fat: 28 g. Protein: 1 g. Carbs: 6 g.

INGREDIENTS

- 300 grams Green Cabbage, shredded
- 100 grams Carrots, cut into thin strips
- 50 grams Crushed Pineapples

For the Dressing:

- 1 cup Sunflower Oil
- 1 tbsp Garlic Powder
- 1 tbsp Onion Powder
- 1 tbsp Flax Seeds
- 1 tbsp Lemon Juice
- ½ tsp Salt
- ¼ tsp Cayenne

DIRECTIONS

1. Combine all ingredients in a food processor. Process until smooth.
2. Toss cabbage, carrots, and pineapples with the prepared dressing.
3. Chill for at least an hour.

86. CURRIED CAULIFLOWER SALAD

Preparation Time: 10 minutes

Cooking Time: 5

Servings: 4

NUTRITIONAL VALUES: Calories: 165 Fat: 14 g. Protein: 3 g. Carbs: 9 g.

INGREDIENTS

- 300 grams Cauliflower, chopped into florets
- 100 grams Cherry Tomatoes
- 150 grams Red Bell Pepper, diced
- 50 grams White Onions, diced
- handful of Fresh Cilantro for garnish

For the Dressing:

- 1/4 cup Olive Oil
- 1 tbsp Lime Juice
- ½ tsp Turmeric Powder
- 1 tbsp Garam Masala
- 2 Green Chilis, minced
- Salt, to taste

DIRECTIONS

1. Blanch cauliflowers in boiling water for 3 minutes. Drain and allow to cool.
2. Whisk all ingredients for the dressing in a bowl. Toss in cauliflower, tomatoes, peppers, and onions.
3. Top with fresh cilantro.

CURRIED CAULIFLOWER SALAD

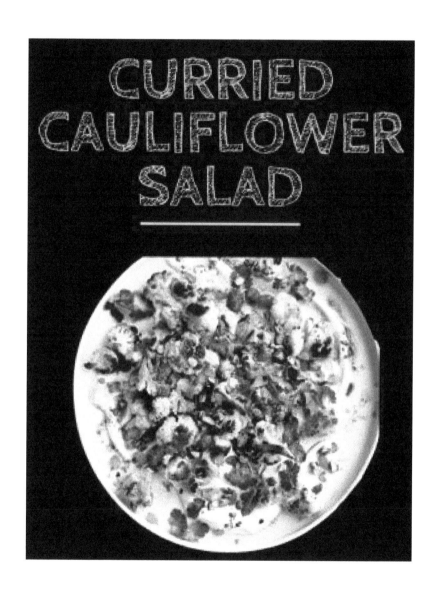

87. ASIAN SLAW AND EDAMAME SALAD

Preparation Time: 5 minutes

Servings: 4

NUTRITIONAL VALUES: Calories: 190 Fat: 16 g. Protein: 3 g. Carbs: 9 g.

INGREDIENTS

- 50 grams Edamame
- 150 grams Carrots, cut into thin strips
- 150 grams Jicama, cut into thin strips
- 1 tbsp Sesame Seeds

For the Dressing:

- 3 tbsp Olive Oil
- 1 tbsp Sesame Oil
- 1 tbsp Tamari
- 1 tbsp Peanut Butter
- 1 tbsp Lime Juice
- 2 Red Chilis, minced
- 1 tbsp Erythritol

DIRECTIONS

1. Whisk all ingredients for the dressing in a bowl.

2. Toss in edamame, carrots, and jicama.

88.   FALAFEL SALAD

Preparation Time: 10 minutes

Servings: 4

NUTRITIONAL VALUES: Calories: 143 Fat: 11 g. Protein: 3 g. Carbs: 9 g.

INGREDIENTS

- 300 grams Romaine Lettuce, chopped
- 50 grams Chickpeas
- 100 grams Tomatoes, diced
- 50 grams Shallots, thinly sliced
- Fresh Parsley for garnish

For the Dressing:

- ¼ cup Vegennaise
- 1 tsp Garlic Powder
- 1 tbsp Lemon Juice
- 1 tsp Cumin Powder
- ¼ tsp Salt

DIRECTIONS

1. Whisk together all ingredients for the dressing in a bowl.
2. Toss in lettuce, chickpeas, shallots, and tomatoes.
3. Top with chopped fresh parsley.

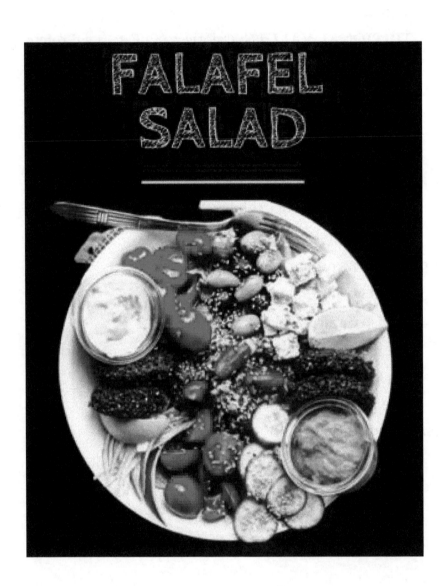

89.   ASIAN AVOCADO SALAD

Preparation Time: 4 hours

Servings: 4

NUTRITIONAL VALUES: Calories: 298 Fat: 29 g. Protein: 3 g. Carbs: 9 g.

INGREDIENTS

- 2 Avocados, peeled and diced
- 1 tbsp Sesame Seeds

For the Dressing:

- ¼ cup Sesame Oil
- 2 tbsp Lime Juice
  - tbsp Tamari
- 1 tbsp Minced Shallots
- 2 Red Chilis, minced
- 1 tbsp Erythritol

DIRECTIONS

1. Whisk all ingredients for the dressing in a bowl.
2. Toss in avocado and top with sesame seeds.

ASIAN AVOCADO SALAD

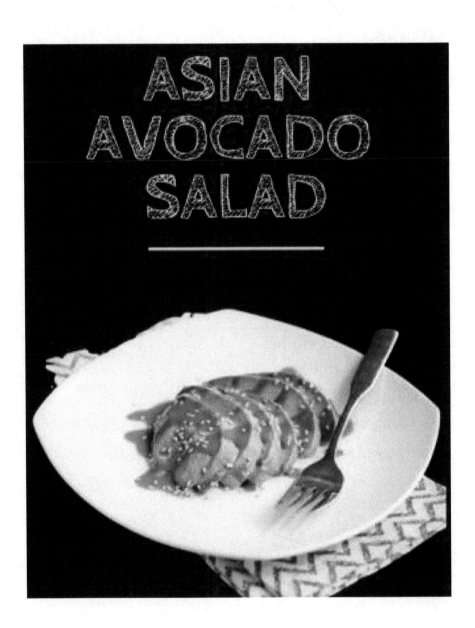

90. <u>STRAWBERRY JAM</u>

Preparation time: 10 minutes

Cooking time: 2 minutes

Servings: 6

INGREDIENTS

- 2 tablespoons chia seeds
- 4 tablespoons stevia
- 2 pounds strawberries, halved

DIRECTIONS

1. In your instant pot, mix stevia with strawberries and chia seeds, stir, cover and cook on High for 2 minutes.
2. Stir again, divide into cups and serve.
3. Enjoy!

NUTRITION VALUES: Calories 110, Fat 2, Fiber 2, Carbs 2, Protein 3

STRAWBERRY JAM

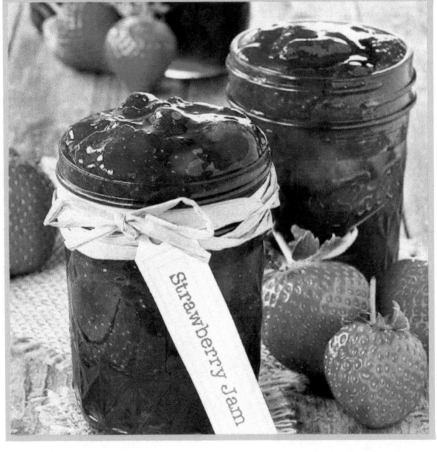

91. POACHED FIGS

Preparation time: 10 minutes

Cooking time: 3 minutes

Servings: 4

INGREDIENTS

- 1 cup red wine
- 1 pound figs
- ½ cup pine nuts
- Stevia to the taste

DIRECTIONS

1. Put the wine in your instant pot, add stevia to the taste, stir well, add steamer basket, add figs inside, cover and cook on Low for 3 minutes.
2. Divide figs into bowls, drizzle wine over them, sprinkle pine nuts at the end and serve.
3. Enjoy!

NUTRITION VALUES: Calories 100, Fat 3, Fiber 1, Carbs 2, Protein 2

Poached
Figs

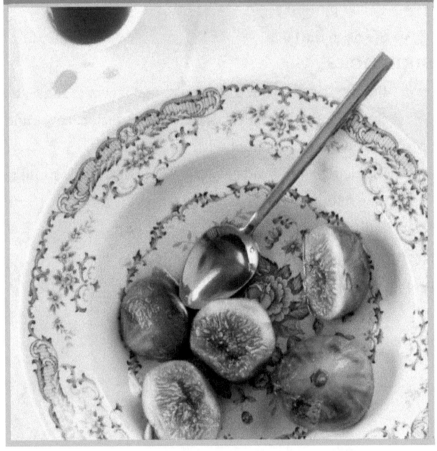

92. MANGO JAM

Preparation time: 10 minutes

Cooking time: 10 minutes

Servings: 8

INGREDIENTS

- 1 and ½ pounds mango, peeled and cubed
- 1 teaspoon nigella seeds
- Stevia to the taste
- ½ cup apple cider vinegar
- 1 inch ginger, grated
- 1 cinnamon stick
- 4 cardamom pods
- 4 cloves

DIRECTIONS

1. In your instant pot, mix mango with nigella seeds, stevia, vinegar, ginger, cinnamon, cardamom and cloves, stir, cover and cook on High for 10 minutes.
2. Stir again, discard cinnamon stick, divide into dessert bowls and serve.
3. Enjoy!

NUTRITION VALUES: Calories 100, Fat 2, Fiber 2, Carbs 2, Protein 3

Mango Jam

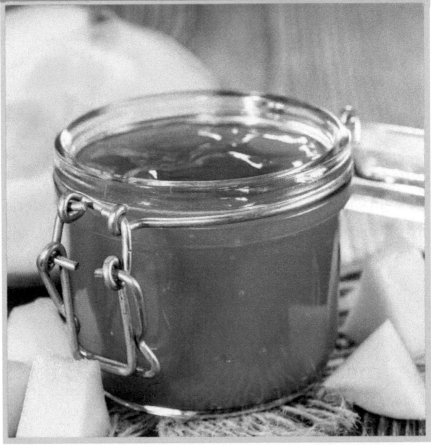

93. RASPBERRY CURD

Preparation time: 10 minutes

Cooking time: 2 minutes

Servings: 4

INGREDIENTS

- 2 tablespoons lemon juice
- 2 tablespoons vegetable oil
- Stevia to the taste
- 12 ounces raspberries
- 2 tablespoons flax meal mixed with 4 tablespoons water

DIRECTIONS

1. In your instant pot, mix raspberries with stevia to the taste, oil, lemon juice and flax meal, stir, cover and cook on High for 2 minutes.
2. Stir well, divide into dessert cups and serve.
3. Enjoy!

NUTRITION VALUES: Calories 111, Fat 3, Fiber 2, Carbs 6, Protein 3

Raspberry Curd

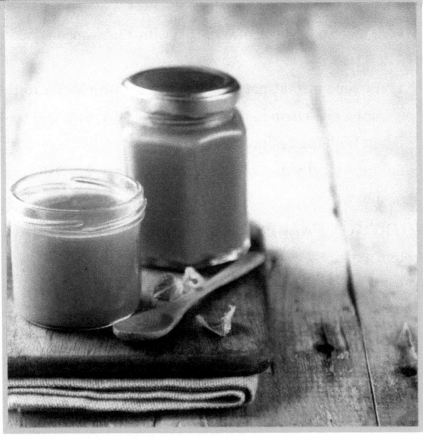

94. **LEMON PUDDING**

Preparation time: 10 minutes

Cooking time: 5 minutes

Servings: 7

INGREDIENTS

- 3 cups coconut milk
- Juice from 2 lemons
- Lemon zest from 2 lemons, grated
- ½ cup maple syrup
- 3 tablespoons coconut oil
- 3 tablespoons flax meal mixed with 6 tablespoons water
- 4 drops lemon oil
- 2 tablespoons gelatin
- 1 cup water

DIRECTIONS

1. In your blender, mix coconut milk with lemon juice, lemon zest, maple syrup, coconut oil, flax meal, lemon oil and gelatin and pulse really well.
2. Divide this into small jars and cover them with their lids.
3. Add the water to your instant pot, add steamer basket, arrange jars inside, cover and cook on High for 5 minutes.
4. Serve puddings cold.
5. Enjoy!

NUTRITION VALUES: Calories 121, Fat 3, Fiber 2, Carbs 6, Protein 4

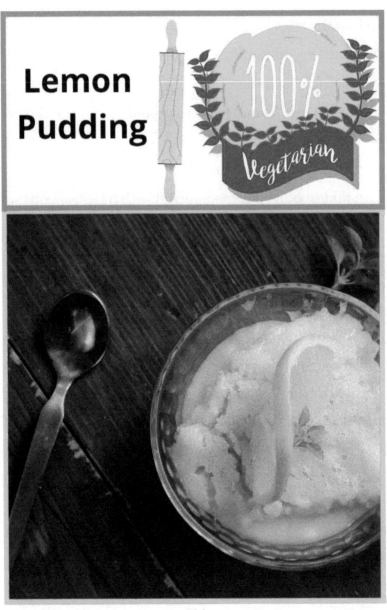

95. PEACHES OATMEAL

Preparation time: 10 minutes

Cooking time: 3 minutes

Servings: 4

INGREDIENTS

- 4 cups water
- 1 peach, chopped
- 2 cups rolled oats
- 1 teaspoon vanilla extract
- 2 tablespoons flax meal
- ½ almonds, chopped

DIRECTIONS

1. In your instant pot, mix water with peach, oats, vanilla extract, flax meal and almonds, stir, cover and cook on High for 3 minutes.
2. Stir again, divide into bowls and serve.
3. Enjoy!

NUTRITION VALUES: Calories 142, Fat 3, Fiber 3, Carbs 7, Protein 4

96. <u>PUMPKIN PUDDING</u>

Preparation time: 10 minutes

Cooking time: 15 minutes

Servings: 6

INGREDIENTS

- 3 cups water
- 1 tablespoon vegetable oil
- 1 cup steel cut oats
- 1 cup pumpkin puree
- ¼ cup maple syrup
- 2 teaspoons cinnamon powder

DIRECTIONS

1. Set your instant pot on sauté mode, add oil, heat it up, add oats, stir and toast them for a couple of minutes.
2. Add pumpkin puree, water, cinnamon and maple syrup, stir, cover the pot, cook on High for 10 minutes, divide into dessert bowls and serve.
3. Enjoy!

NUTRITION VALUES: Calories 212, Fat 5, Fiber 5, Carbs 27, Protein 5

97.   FRUITS PIE

Preparation time: 10 minutes

Cooking time: 10 minutes

Servings: 4

INGREDIENTS

- 1 plum, chopped
- 1 pear, chopped
- 1 apple, chopped
- 2 tablespoons stevia
- 1 cup water
- ¼ cup coconut, shredded
- ½ teaspoon cinnamon powder
- 3 tablespoons coconut oil
- ¼ cup pecans, chopped

DIRECTIONS

1. Put plum, apple and pear in a heatproof bowl, add coconut oil, coconut, cinnamon and stevia and toss to coat.
2. Add water to your instant pot, add steamer basket, add bowl inside, cover, cook on High for 10 minutes, divide into bowls and serve with pecans on top.
3. Enjoy!

NUTRITION VALUES: Calories 152, Fat 4, Fiber 4, Carbs 14, Protein 7

98. <u>POMEGRANATE PUDDING</u>

Preparation time: 5 minutes

Cooking time: 2 minutes

Servings: 2

INGREDIENTS

- 1 cup steel cut oats
- 1 cup water
- ¾ cup pomegranate juice
- Seeds from 1 pomegranate

DIRECTIONS

1. In your instant pot, mix oats with water, pomegranate juice and pomegranate seeds, stir, cover and cook on High for 2 minutes.
2. Divide into dessert bowls and serve cold.
3. Enjoy!

NUTRITION VALUES: Calories 212, Fat 4, Fiber 5, Carbs 20, Protein 5

99. BANANA CAKE

Preparation time: 10 minutes

Cooking time: 1 hour

Servings: 4

INGREDIENTS

- 1 cup water
- 1 and ½ cups coconut stevia
- 2 cups coconut flour
- 3 bananas, peeled and mashed
- 2 tablespoons flax meal mixed with 4 tablespoons water
- 2 teaspoon baking powder
- 1 teaspoon cinnamon powder
- 1 teaspoon nutmeg powder

DIRECTIONS

1. In a bowl, mix flax meal with sugar, baking powder, cinnamon, nutmeg, banana and flour, stir well, pour into a greased cake pan and cover with tin foil.
2. Add the water to your instant pot, add steamer basket, and cake pan, cover and cook on High for 1 hour.
3. Slice, divide on dessert plates and serve.
4. Enjoy!

NUTRITION VALUES: Calories 326 Fat 11 Fiber 1.1 Carbs 55 Protein 4.3

Banana Cake

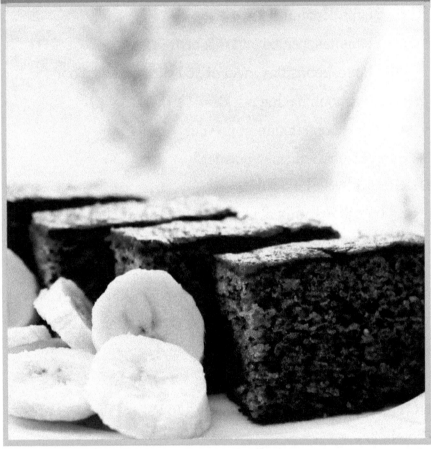

100. BUFFALO TOFU PINWHEELS

Preparation Time: 20 minutes

Servings: 45 pinwheels

INGREDIENTS

- 3 green onions thinly sliced
- 6-oz. light cream cheese softened
- ½ cup Frank's Red-hot sauce
- 8-oz. sliced tofu medallions
- 4-6 strips of bread shaped like thin logs

DIRECTIONS

1. Mix your tofu with your cream cheese, green onions, and hot sauce until well blended.

2. Spread the buffalo tofu on the bread thin logs and roll them up like a jelly roll. Cut into ½ inch slices, place them in the fridge to chill.

3. Garnish with some sliced green onions.

BUFFALO TOFU PINWHEELS

101. VEGETARIAN COCONUT LIME NOODLES

Preparation Time: 35 minutes

Servings: 4

INGREDIENTS

- ½ tsp ground or fresh grated ginger
- 1 can full fat coconut milk
- 4 tbsp sesame seeds
- 2 packages of shirataki noodles
- Juice and zest of 1 lime

Optional:

- Red pepper flakes
- Salt

DIRECTIONS

1. Drain and rinse your noodles and place them in a pot over a temperature of medium heat, adding in the ingredients listed above. Mix them well to combine all the ingredients.

2. Next, place a lid on the pot, partially covering the pot, and cook the noodles for 10 minutes.

3. Next, lower your heat to low, continuing to cook for an additional 10 minutes.

4. Once your noodles are done, garnish them with whatever vegetables or tofu you would like to add to them.

VEGETARIAN COCONUT LIME NOODLES

102. SWEET AND SOUR CUCUMBER NOODLES WITH SOBA

Preparation Time: 35 minutes

Servings: 4

INGREDIENTS

- 2-3 Cucumbers medium
- 2 tsp. Honey
- ½ cup Rice Vinegar
- 4-oz. Soba Noodles
- 1 tbsp. Soy sauce

Optional:

- Green onions
- Sriracha sauce
- Hot sauce
- Sesame seeds
- Sambal olek

DIRECTIONS

1. Cook your Soba in some boiling water for only 5 minutes. They should be undercooked. Once done, drain them and rinse.
2. Combine your noodles with soy sauce and set them aside.
3. Now using a julienne peeler, thinly slice the cucumbers so that they are noodle-like.
4. Next, in a large bowl, add in your rice vinegar and honey, whisking till blended well.

5. Now, coat your cucumber noodles with the dressing and chill for 30 minutes.
6. Blend the soba with the cucumber and serve!

103. FRIED GOAT CHEESE

Preparation Time: 30 minutes

Servings: 2

INGREDIENTS

- 2 tbsp poppy seeds
- 2 tbsp sesame seeds
- 1 tsp onion flakes
- 4 -oz. goat cheese cut into ½ inch thick medallions
- 1 tsp garlic flakes

DIRECTIONS

1. Cut the goat cheese into ½ inch thick medallions.
2. Place the poppy seeds, garlic, onion, and sesame seeds in a bowl and mix well.
3. Place the goat cheese into the bowl individually and coat each side with seasoning.
4. Using a skillet with some olive oil for non-sticking, heat the pan to medium heat.
5. Fry the goat cheese on each side, making sure they do not fully melt.
6. Place on a plate for serving.

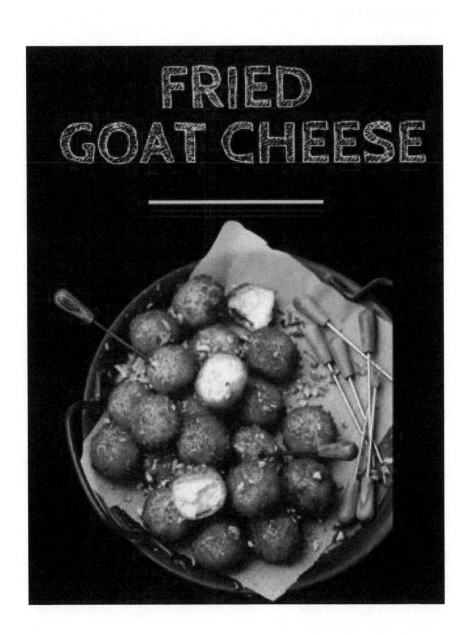

FRIED
GOAT CHEESE

104. ORANGE MINT JALAPENO SALAD

Preparation Time: 10 minutes

Servings: 4

INGREDIENTS

- 10 assorted oranges
- Olive oil
- ¼ cup pine nuts
- 2 tbsp chopped jalapeno
- 1 handful of fresh mint leaves finely chopped

Optional: Sea salt

DIRECTIONS

1. Heat a small pan to a temperature of medium heat and sauté the pine nuts until golden brown. This should be about 2 minutes. They should be fragrant.
2. Place them on a cutting board using a knife to cut the ends off the oranges and slice the skin off. Cutting each orange into slices discard the orange seeds.
3. Arrange your slices on a plate and top it with chopped mint, jalapeno and pine nuts. Sprinkle with salt if you like and drizzle with olive oil for taste.
4. Serve immediately.

ORANGE MINT JALAPENO SALAD

105. BROCCOLI SALAD

Preparation Time: 15 minutes

Servings: 1-2

INGREDIENTS

- ½ cup shredded carrots
- ¼ cup raw sunflower seeds
- ½ cup red onions
- 1 head of broccoli cut into bite size pieces

Optional:

- ¼ cup raisins
- Sea salt
- Pepper

DIRECTIONS

1. In a bowl, add in the carrots, broccoli, red onion, sunflower seeds, and raisins if you like. Use any dressing that you like or the one mentioned below and toss it until the ingredients are evenly coated.
2. Serve and enjoy!

BROCCOLI SALAD

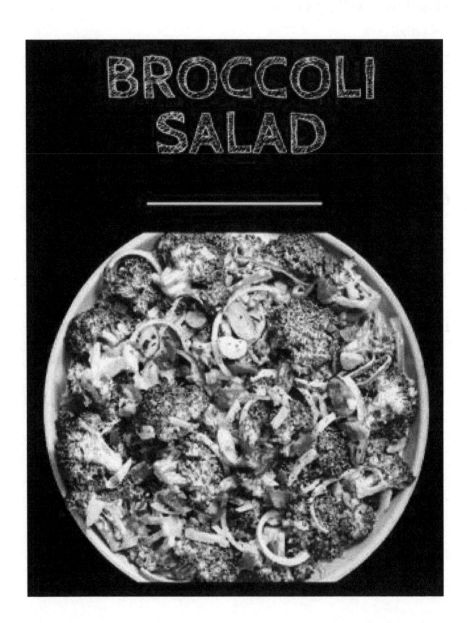

106. RHUBARB AND STRAWBERRY DESSERT

Preparation time: 10 minutes

Cooking time: 10 minutes

Servings: 4

INGREDIENTS

- 1/3 cup water
- 2 pound rhubarb, roughly chopped
- 3 tablespoons stevia
- 1 pound strawberries, halved
- A few mint leaves, chopped

DIRECTIONS

1. In your instant pot, mix water with rhubarb, stevia and strawberries, stir a bit, cover and cook on High for 10 minutes.
2. Add mint, stir, leave aside compote for a few minutes, divide into cups and serve.
3. Enjoy!

NUTRITION VALUES: Calories 100, Fat 2, Fiber 2, Carbs 3, Protein 2

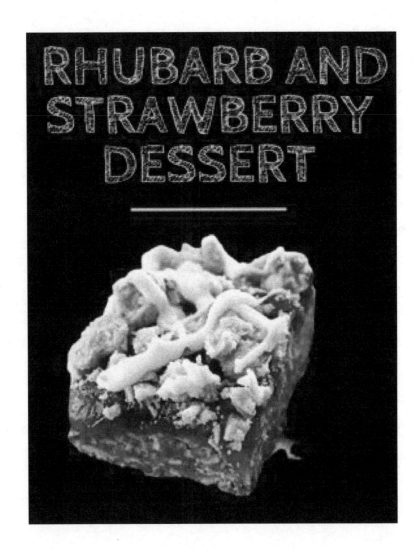

RHUBARB AND STRAWBERRY DESSERT

Recipe

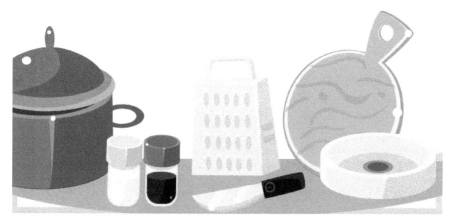

CONCLUSION

Thanks for reading this guide. It is likewise important for you to have a goal. One goal is enough. Several short-term goals may also work for you – anything doable will do. Set realistic goals for yourself and stick to them. For instance, would you want to be vegetarian for only a week? Or would you want to have a one-month trial period? It is advisable that you don't do anything drastic, as it's so easy to backslide and lose the drive. It would also help to decide on the type of vegetarian you want to be.

As a beginner to vegetarianism, you may be tempted to purchase ready-to-eat meals, which companies claim as vegetarian. Most of these meals have been prepared with a set of calories in mind. You may choose to just have these meals delivered, though they may get expensive in the long run. Thus, maintaining this lifestyle depends on how much you are willing to spend. Should you buy your meals, choose a good vegetarian restaurant.

Another option is to research on various vegetarian recipes. Many are available online, and they have been prepared by chefs and food experts. Meanwhile, expand your search by adding a certain cuisine. Look for Japanese vegetarian recipes, Chinese, Mediterranean, or Middle Eastern.

Though risky, you may also up your ante and invent your recipes. You may substitute vegetables and fruits for variation. For example, you could have oatmeal with bananas on Monday, then oatmeal mixed with whole grain cereal and blueberries on Tuesday.

Lightning Source UK Ltd.
Milton Keynes UK
UKHW021820160421
382091UK00005B/98